Decolonial Care

Critical Caribbean Studies

Series Editors: Yolanda Martínez-San Miguel, Carter Mathes, and Kathleen López

Editorial Board: Carlos U. Decena, Rutgers University; Alex Dupuy, Wesleyan University; Aisha Khan, New York University; April J. Mayes, Pomona College; Patricia Mohammed, University of West Indies; Martin Munro, Florida State University; F. Nick Nesbitt, Princeton University; Michelle Stephens, Rutgers University; Deborah Thomas, University of Pennsylvania; and Lanny Thompson, University of Puerto Rico

Focused particularly in the twentieth and twenty-first centuries, although attentive to the context of earlier eras, this series encourages interdisciplinary approaches and methods and is open to scholarship in a variety of areas, including anthropology, cultural studies, diaspora and transnational studies, environmental studies, gender and sexuality studies, history, and sociology. The series pays particular attention to the four main research clusters of Critical Caribbean Studies at Rutgers University, where the coeditors serve as members of the executive board: Caribbean Critical Studies Theory and the Disciplines; Archipelagic Studies and Creolization; Caribbean Aesthetics, Poetics, and Politics; and Caribbean Colonialities.

For a complete list of titles in the series, please see the last page of the book.

Decolonial Care

~

Reimagining Caregiving in the French Caribbean

JENNIFER BOUM MAKE

Rutgers University Press
New Brunswick, Camden, and Newark, New Jersey
London and Oxford

Rutgers University Press is a department of Rutgers, The State University of New Jersey, one of the leading public research universities in the nation. By publishing worldwide, it furthers the University's mission of dedication to excellence in teaching, scholarship, research, and clinical care.

978-1-9788-4045-4 (cloth)
978-1-9788-4044-7 (paper)
978-1-9788-4046-1 (epub)

Cataloging-in-publication data is available from the Library of Congress.
LCCN 2024049535

A British Cataloging-in-Publication record for this book is available from the British Library.

Copyright © 2025 by Jennifer Boum Make
All rights reserved

No part of this book may be reproduced or utilized in any form or by any means, electronic or mechanical, or by any information storage and retrieval system, without written permission from the publisher. Please contact Rutgers University Press, 106 Somerset Street, New Brunswick, NJ 08901. The only exception to this prohibition is "fair use" as defined by U.S. copyright law.

References to internet websites (URLs) were accurate at the time of writing. Neither the author nor Rutgers University Press is responsible for URLs that may have expired or changed since the manuscript was prepared.

∞ The paper used in this publication meets the requirements of the American National Standard for Information Sciences—Permanence of Paper for Printed Library Materials, ANSI Z39.48-1992.

rutgersuniversitypress.org

For Maman

Contents

	Introduction	1
1.	Curating Silences	27
2.	Voices of the BUMIDOM, or the Colonial Legacy of Care Work	57
3.	Inhabiting the Land after Environmental Damage	89
4.	Rebellious Care, or Deconstructing the Myth of the *Poto-mitan* Woman	119
	Coda	145
	Acknowledgments	161
	Notes	165
	References	187
	Notes on Cover Art	201
	Index	203

Decolonial Care

Introduction

This book is an invitation to think about care *decolonially* from the outside of coloniality. It proposes a situated critical interrogation about the ways dynamics of caregiving have been shaped by the enduring legacies of French colonialism and slavery in the French Caribbean. Ultimately though, its aim is to revitalize practices of care from the overseas territories of Guadeloupe and Martinique in foregrounding how these practices are imagined anew through a variety of media (novels, graphic narratives, and curatorial discourse). To set the tone for our discussion, let's be traversed by the words of James Baldwin, who urges us to face our history as a path forward: "To accept one's past—one's history—is not the same thing as drowning in it; it is learning how to use it" ([1963] 2013, 157). Let us also be inspired by Stéphane Dufoix, who encourages us to engage in the work of decolonizing our attitudes, thoughts, and methods: "'Décoloniser' n'est pas un mot diabolique. C'est un mot plein d'espoir pour qui sait y saisir les promesses qu'il engage" ("To decolonize" is not a diabolical word. It is a word filled with hope for who knows how to grasp the promises it involves) (2023, 92–93).[1]

Care: A Definition

Turning to the definition of the term, we find it is synonymous with "attention, carefulness, precision, meticulousness, mindfulness, responsibility, conscientiousness, kindness, solicitude, lovingness, and concern," among others.[2] In short, following Joan

Tronto and Berenice Fisher's expansive definition, "caring [is] viewed as species activity that includes everything that we do to maintain, continue, and repair our 'world' so we can live in it as well as possible" (1990, 40). However, what the word conceals at first glance is the historically unfair distribution of the responsibilities for care. In fact, since the 1980s when the field of care studies first emerged in North America, theorists of care made it a point to make visible primarily the gendered division of caring, whether unpaid or underpaid, as well as its systemic and systematic devaluation.

In her 1982 seminal work, *In a Different Voice*, American psychologist Carol Gilligan, having interviewed women and girls to study their moral development and conception of morality, argues that "the expression of care is seen as the fulfillment of [their] moral responsibility" (73). This is not to support an essentialized distribution of the exercise of care along gender lines but rather to attest to the deep-seated feminization of care. One that reinforces the relegation of caring responsibilities to women and girls, whether in domestic settings—such as home maintenance or child-rearing—or in caregiving professions. Following Gilligan's study, this socially constructed feminine orientation toward care stands in contrast with "the formal logic of fairness that informs the justice approach," typically associated with men's moral judgment (73)—the latter being valorized over the devaluation and marginalization of dispositions to care.

Seen through the lens of Gilligan, care is primarily defined against the backdrop of gendered socialization. A framework that theorists like Joan Tronto (1993), Evelyn Nakano Glenn (2012, 2000), Pascale Molinier, Sandra Laugier, and Patricia Paperman (2009), Pascale Molinier (2013), Sandra Laugier (2021), and Fabienne Brugère ([2011] 2021), among others, have expanded to include that care is not only gendered but also racialized and class based. In *Moral Boundaries: A Political Argument for an Ethic of Care* (1993), Tronto observes, for example, that "care has mainly been the work of slaves, servants, and women in Western history" (113). In *Qu'est-ce que le care? Souci des autres, sensibilité et responsabilité* (2009), Molinier, Laugier, and Paperman similarly insist on the fact that "ceux/celles à qui l'on avait *déjà* refusé les droits d'une citoyenneté pleine et entière, en l'occurrence les esclaves, les travailleurs engagés sous contrat ('indentured workers'), les sujets colonisés, les immigrés et les femmes, ont été reléguées aux tâches de *care*" (care tasks have been relegated to those who had *already* been denied the rights to full citizenship, specifically slaves, indentured workers, immigrants, and women) (117). Here, categories of individuals are amalgamated to form the group of "subalterns" that Brugère identifies in *L'éthique du care* (2011) as the caregiving labor force *par excellence*.

Revisiting this original categorization of the distribution of caregivers, *Decolonial Care* directs attention toward the interplay of racialization, gender dynamics, and class disparities intrinsic to the history of colonialism and enslavement, spanning from "hexagonal" (i.e., metropolitan) France to the French Caribbean. In the historical context of exploitative care within Francophone cultures, we can already discern the visual representation of racialized and gendered caregiving. For instance, we encounter the depiction of the Black nanny in artworks such as Édouard Manet's *Enfants aux Tuileries* (circa 1861–1862) or the exoticized Black maidservant portrayed in Jean-Léon Gérôme's *Bain turc ou maure (deux femmes)* (1872).

Caribbean fiction in French is also populated by women caregivers in public or domestic spheres. For instance, to name a few, in Haitian writer Jacques Roumain's *Gouverneurs de la Rosée* ([1944] 2004), the mother (Délira) and the wife (Annaïse) serve the role of unflinching advocates to Manuel, the self-sacrificing male hero of the Fonds-Rouge community. In *La Rue Cases-Nègres* ([1950] 2000) by Martinican writer Joseph Zobel, we meet José Hassam's hard-working and devoted grandmother (M'man Tine) who works in horrid conditions cutting sugarcane for a *béké* owner to build a future away from the plantation for her grandson.[3] The figure of the benevolent grandmother (and abused wife to Asdrubal) is present also in Guadeloupean writer Gisèle Pineau's *L'exil selon Julia*

([1996] 2000) where her son Maréchal denies her the choice to stay in her beloved Guadeloupe. On all counts, "Caribbean women have been configured in regional fiction as infinitely willing and expected to orient themselves in service to communities [or partners, children, and aging parents] that are little attentive to their individual needs and desires" (Glover 2021, 17). Reproductive work, or, more precisely exploitative care work clearly appears here as being racialized, gendered, and socially as well as culturally inherited.

More specific to the inside of colonial enslavement, the activities that define care are a commodified resource; and the existence of caregivers is thereby incorporated into colonial exploitation, or what French political scientist and historian Françoise Vergès terms "an economy of exhaustion" (2019a)—a direct result of the extraction of labor. As part of the plantation system in the then official French colonies of Guadeloupe and Martinique, the enslaved were working the land and were incorporated within the domestic sphere acting as caregivers, nurturing and caring for the master's family and maintaining the household (see the definition of the analytical concept of the "Plantationocene" and the way it shapes extractive relations to human and nonhuman bodies in the work of Anna Tsing [2015], Donna Haraway [2015], or Malcolm Ferdinand [2019], among others). On the colonial plantation, "Black women's wombs," Vergès also reminds us, "were made into capital and their children were transformed into currency," following the *Code Noir* of 1685 (2019a). The coercive and extractive practices that support the organization of work on the colonial plantation mean that daily activities that maintain life—in short, "free" labor—become colonized acts of caring.

COLONIZED CARING, OR THE PRODUCTION OF UNCARING IN FRENCH CARIBBEAN CONTEXTS

Through this, my approach underscores the dialectical relation between the amplification of care on one end and its absence, denial, or depletion on the other—caring and uncaring, to not care, thereby emerging as two sides of the same coin. In fact, prolonged and extensive practices of neglect toward human and nonhuman lives have come to define the relationship between hexagonal France and its overseas territories well beyond the "end" of formal colonial rule. To Aimé Césaire's point in 1967, twenty-one years after the law of departmentalization that gave the same administrative status as mainland departments to the former colonies of Guadeloupe and Martinique alongside French Guiana, Mayotte, and Réunion,[4] "les Antillais ne savent pas s'ils sont des Français à part entière, mais ils savent qu'ils sont des Français entièrement à part" (Antilleans do not know if they are fully French, but they know that they are entirely separate French).[5] Similar to Aimé Césaire, Vergès notes there is "[un] écart entre territoire hexagonal et territoire extra-hexagonal (donc pas tout à fait 'national')" (a gap between the hexagonal territory and extra-hexagonal territory [therefore not quite "national"]), suggesting that in the French national imagination there is a unique historical and cultural distinction established between hexagonal France and France's overseas territories—a distinction that has throughout history been used to pass off as acceptable what happens outside the Hexagon (2011, 81–82).

The multifaceted dimensions of such organized uncaring well beyond the "ends" of France's colonial rule become, for example, manifest in the usage of chlordecone, a toxic and highly persistent pesticide, in banana plantations in Guadeloupe and Martinique between the years 1972 and 1993—all the while being banned by the U.S. Environmental Protection Agency in 1976 and ruled carcinogenic in 1979 by the International Agency for Research on Cancer. First brought to the public's attention in the 2007 exposé *Chronique d'un empoisonnement annoncé* (Chronicle of a poisoning foretold) by Martinican intellectuals Louis Boutrin and Raphaël Confiant, the pesticide used to eradicate the banana weevil, or *charançon*, is known to have permanently contaminated the islands' soils and sources of potable water, jeopardizing the habitability of these territories. Today this issue is also in part responsible for water insecurity in the region. In February 2024, the umbrella organization Lyannaj kont' pwofitasyon (Collective against Outrageous Exploitation)[6] demonstrated against the French government's inaction amid the water crisis in Guadeloupe, condemning "l'irresponsabilité, le mépris et la mise en danger de la vie des Guadeloupéens par les autorités françaises" (the irresponsibility, contempt, and endangerment of the lives of Guadeloupeans by the French authorities) (Lebastard 2024)—a striking allusion to the enduring repercussions of neglect on those living in contaminated territories.

In another vein, we see the asymmetrical burden of caregiving on populations from the French Caribbean expressed in Martinican writer Françoise Ega's 1978 novel *Lettres à une Noire: Récit antillais* (Letters to a Black woman: an Antillean story). The narrative features a collection of fictional letters in which Ega tells about the lives of women who have emigrated from the French Caribbean to mainland France in the 1960s to become live-in maids in predominantly white, bourgeois families. There, they clean, cook, and take care of children—in other words, they attend to the personal needs of others. After seeking a job as a household worker, Ega investigates what she describes as a "new Black slave trade" (80, translation mine).

Ega's careful report on the lives of those she calls her "sisters" draws attention to the interconnection between the burden of care and socioeconomic exploitation. If, as regards the law of departmentalization, Guadeloupeans and Martinicans were "theoretically bestowed the same rights and privileges [as] any other French citizens" (10), scholar Adlai Murdoch notes in the introduction to his edited volume *The Struggle of Non-Sovereign Caribbean Territories* (2021), the inequalities of coloniality whereby "an extended and repeated pattern of economic exploitation in which external influences use local labor simply as an expendable means to a profitable end" were consolidated (42). For what these accounts of uncaring ultimately reveal is that practices of care enmeshed in coloniality are not so caring and do harm, using the intrinsic invisibility of care to further dependency, exploitation, and marginalization.

VISIBLE, BUT VOICELESS?

Considering the specificities of the exercise of caring, French psychologist Pascale Molinier describes these types of activity as "savoir-faire discrets" (discreet *savoir-faire* [pl.]) (2006, 343), highlighting their constitutive invisibility. For Molinier concludes, "Le travail de care se voit avant tout quand il échoue" (Care work is above all seen when it fails) (344). Caring, therefore, is deemed essential for maintaining life yet often goes widely unnoticed and unacknowledged. Central to the work of care theorists then is the struggle for visibility—which Laugier identifies in efforts "to make either oppression or those who are oppressed visible" (2021, 62). Tellingly, *The Care Manifesto*, published by the Care Collective in 2020 in the midst of the COVID-19 pandemic, opens with the following statement: "Our world is one in which carelessness reigns" (1). At a time during which the vital importance but devaluation of care workers in our everyday lives became evident to all, the authors of *The Care Manifesto* strongly advocated for addressing a blatant deficit in care—that is, in their words, "prioritizing the needs of those who have been most marginalized, violated and negated by uncaring nation states" (60).

In point of fact, this is where theorists of care locate an ethic of care through which the values of caring are no longer excluded from public consideration but are instead re-empowered to start penetrating the political so as to achieve a more just society, to "involve the relatively disenfranchised in the political world," to borrow from the Care Collective. I believe here that positionality must be considered as part of the reorganization of the landscape of care. In other words, where do the aspirations for a "truly" caring world originate? Can such a world take hold on the foundations of carelessness, and under what conditions? Who allows greater visibility as part of existing uncaring social structures? And finally, must those whose lives are currently marginalized wait until caring states or economies come into existence? This is obviously not to dismiss calls for attention to what is here but not seen, which an ethic of care supports—what Laugier effectively terms "a simple will to *see the visible*" (2021, 67, emphasis in original). Rather, considering the impact of carelessness in the context of the French Caribbean, I am interested in an examination of practices of refusal of uncaring, fueling radical imaginaries of caregiving.

Decolonizing Care

Central to *Decolonial Care* is looking at how care comes to be defined, manipulated, and grappled with in attempts to decolonize, to disentangle, or "delink" (Mignolo and Walsh 2018, 106) it from its colonial heritage. The ways relations of care have arisen in the context of the French Caribbean and in relation to hexagonal France have resulted in patterns of exploitation that continually endanger the well-being of human and nonhuman lives and habitats. Studying the kind of care that emerges from the condition of enduring violence, French scholar Elsa Dorlin proposes the concept of "dirty care," emphasizing forms of attention to others that result from the constant threat of the destruction of one's existence. The need to care thus understood is "negative" for it means to live like prey and be continually on one's guard—it means being "concerned for others, in order to anticipate what they want, will, or can *do to us*—which might devalue, exhaust, insult, isolate, injure, worry, deny, frighten, or de-realize us" (155, emphasis in original). This kind of attention paid to others takes shape out of concern for one's own survival, "aris[ing] within and by means of violence" (154). As such, Dorlin helps us think about the forms of concern for others that come out of a social system traversed by violence; care here means not to take care or take responsibility for the self and others but rather to invalidate the self for it is constrained and defined by the necessity to avoid the persecutors or, alternatively, prepare for conflict. For the oppressed, then, maintaining life in repressive contexts, after Tronto and Fisher's definition, means maintaining safety.

Given the circumstances where coerced attention has regressed into a form of "negative care," the decolonial option is useful as regards the possibility to reorient practices of care—reorienting both in the sense of a changing focus, from those who abuse to those subject to abuse, as well as in the sense of reinventing and reimagining, or at least betting on what Argentine scholar Walter Mignolo terms "the decolonial option." In *On Decoloniality* (2018), Mignolo and scholar Catherine Walsh develop decoloniality as a project that implies "epistemic disobedience," for it means "to delink from the colonial matrix of power in order to imagine and engage in becoming decolonial subjects" (125). This work of delinking contains the possibility for retrieving the values of care, such as attentiveness, concern, and responsibility for both the self and others, and attempting to care differently and thus allowing practices of care to not be strictly defined by the leftover impact of colonial oppression and slavery. This means not to dismiss the colonial continuities in the organization and perpetuation of oppressive practices of care but rather to seek to reclaim care by way of decolonizing it, emancipating the praxis from how it was dictated, defined, and distributed by dominant groups.

To do so, *Decolonial Care* investigates decolonized kinds of care from the perspective of those who live with the impact of uncaring, placing the French Caribbean at the center of the reimagining and reconfiguring of practices of care. In this book, I use the terms "decolonial," "decolonize," and "decolonization" in relation to care and in the context of the French Caribbean, for such an approach presses us to consider what caring entails after the damage has been done, while also attending to processes of recovery, reappropriation, and reinvention. Turning to Eve Tuck and K. Wayne Yang's essay "Decolonization Is Not a Metaphor," we are cautioned against the risk of 'killing' the process of decolonization when the latter gets lost in metaphor. They stress, "It is not a philanthropic process of 'helping' the at-risk and alleviating suffering; it is not a generic term for struggle against oppressive conditions and outcomes. The broad umbrella of social justice may have room underneath for all of these efforts. By contrast, *decolonization specifically requires the repatriation of Indigenous land and life*. Decolonization is not a metonym for social justice" (21, emphasis mine).

In *Decolonial Care*, the focus on narratives that engage the territories of Guadeloupe and Martinique in the context of their broader Black Atlantic history is one that precisely supports the revival of an elsewhere from which to creatively remodel an ethic of care. This project refrains from making absolving gestures because it diverges from the rhetoric of care that acknowledges collective failure toward "the vulnerable, the poor, and the weak," as articulated, for instance, in the Care Collective's *The Care Manifesto* (2020, 1). Thereby, it seeks to avoid the possibly vertical positioning that advocates for the prioritization of those who have been most brutalized to instead "repatriate" the question of care to the French Caribbean. "Doubout pou la vi" (Stand up for life), we hear in a promotional video by Lyannaj pou dépolyé Matinik (Collective to Depollute Martinique), calling on the people of both Guadeloupe and Martinique to mobilize against the effects of chlordecone poisoning.[7] In these words ("Doubout pou la vi") there is the expression of finding the means to sustain life, to define care for the self and others in territories impacted by wide-ranging neglect. This does not free from responsibility those accountable for uncaring, but it momentarily grants them less attention. It is thus about reclaiming the narratives of caregiving, shifting the imaginaries on where and to whom care is directed. Through these narratives that center the territories of Guadeloupe and Martinique, in the broader Black Atlantic context, I contend it is possible to imagine new and radically different practices of care in the present.

Caregiving in Texts

Often, care is primarily described as the relationship between mother and child. Many theorists of care, like Tronto (1993), Glenn

(2000), and Molinier, Laugier, and Paperman (2009), have criticized the tendency to oversimplify care relations by exclusively focusing on the mother–child dyad. By privileging this particular dyadic relationship, they observe a potential danger of obscuring the labor involved in care by attributing it solely to maternal love (thus viewed as "women's natural vocation"; Glenn 2000, 87). There is thus the risk to conceal care work behind the naturalization of maternal love, creating the illusion of "unlimited availability" that "underpin[s] the requests made by beneficiaries of care to its purveyors" (Molinier 2012, 301). As such, motherhood is understood as a site of oppression, whereby the capacity for care has been naturalized and exploited. This is not a new way of looking at motherhood, and fictional narratives have played a role in questioning, if not refusing, this naturalization of maternal identity as care usually found in the heteronormative and patriarchal script of mothering.[8]

In fact, in fictional narratives engaging slavery and its enduring legacy in Caribbean contexts, a prevalent literary motif is the rejection of motherhood—for example, in the form of infanticide. This motif exemplifies the refusal to endorse or perpetuate a system that subjected women's bodies and that of their children to enslavement and exploitation. Specific to the act of infanticide in "le roman féminin antillais" (Antillean novels by women), scholar Antoinette Marie Sol comments on its historical ambivalence looking at "les deux faces de l'infanticide" (the two sides of infanticide)—an act led, on the one hand, by "l'amour (épargner un être cher et innocent des horreurs de la servitude)" (love [sparing a loved and innocent one from the horrors of enslavement]), and on the other by "la haine (du système esclavagiste, du maître, de soi)" (hatred [of the slave system, of the master, of oneself]) (2008, 972).

Within the historical framework of colonial enslavement, the act of infanticide can be interpreted as liberating, as depicted by Sol. In fiction, this perspective is illustrated in Haitian writer Evelyne Trouillot's debut novel *Rosalie l'infâme* (2003), set in the French colony of Saint-Domingue (present-day Haiti) during the mid-eighteenth century. In *Rosalie*, Brigitte, the great-aunt of Lisette, the main protagonist, is depicted as drawing inspiration from an Arada midwife who revealed a rope necklace adorned with knots during her trial, each representing one of the seventy babies she had killed at birth. In fact, in the novel's afterword, Trouillot quotes directly the woman's explanation, as it appears in *Antilles 1789: La révolution aux caraïbes* (Abenon and Cauna 1989): "Pour enlever ces jeunes êtres à un honteux esclavage, je plongeais à l'instant de leur naissance une épingle dans leur cerveau par la fontanelle" (To remove these young creatures from the shameful institution of slavery, I inserted a needle in their brain through the fontanel in the moment of their birth) (Trouillot 2003, 139). Given this, the midwife's actions constitute a defiance against gendered violence, disrupting the exploitation of motherhood and reproduction by preventing the children of others from being born into slavery.

In this body of literature, we also see the motif of infanticide directly challenging the mother–child relationship through the act of parents killing their own child. In Haitian-born writer Marie-Célie Agnant's *Le livre d'Emma* (2002), Flore, a young woman of Haitian heritage working in Montréal as an interpreter, meets Emma Bratte, a woman confined to a psychiatric ward after being accused of the murder of her daughter, Lola. Throughout the novel, Emma will not say much about the killing of her daughter, only that through this brutal act she took an already forsaken life ("condamnée" [condemned], 162), a life irremediably enmeshed with personal and collective historical trauma—that of the transatlantic slave trade. Particularly, "la malédiction du sang" (the curse of blood) to which Emma refers invokes the transmission of a genealogy of violence, suffering, and abandonment inscribed into women's bodies. Here, I suggest that the infanticide committed by Emma can be understood, within the context of colonial enslavement and its legacy, as a rebellious act against the inescapability of an interminable past. Through this repeated motif of infanticide, we see the possibility through narratives to articulate the primary refusal of oppression that the mother–child dyad constitutes specifically in the context of the history of enslavement and colonialism in the Caribbean and its legacy.

Building upon the literary expressions that confront care exploitation within the fundamental mother–child dyad in Caribbean contexts, my work in *Decolonial Care* brings together a variety of texts, novels, graphic narratives, and curatorial discourse that all grapple with and are committed to divesting from the legacy of colonialism in practices of care. That is, I propose throughout this book to center narratives that engage with the tension between the inescapability of colonial damage and the possibility of reimagining caregiving in the present and for the future. In care studies there is a focus on the role of literature to interrogate and shape caring practices, considering specifically the strategies and aesthetics that support the remediation of caregiving in literary forms.[9] Through this, it is understood that literature could serve as the locus for the reimagining and restructuring of care practices that have gone rogue, as they have come to define, in the context of this study, exploitative dynamics between the colonizer and the colonized.

As regards the intersection of care and literature, scholars Loïc Bourdeau, Natalie Edwards, and Steven Wilson in their opening essay to the co-edited special issue "The Care (Re)turn in French and Francophone Studies" (2020) engage with Alexandre Gefen's literary study *Réparer le monde: La littérature française face au 21ème siècle* (2018), arguing that "in making 'visible' the destiny of fragile individuals in a world full of challenges" there is the possibility to reorient or redress our attention (2020, 291).[10] More with regard to the (neo)colonial forces driving erasure, dispossession, and dehumanization, it is true that exploring care and the caregiving role in and through literature allows us to investigate the literary attempts that "provide witness to a suppressed historical presence" (Chancy 1997, 13). "Littératures de témoignage" or "testimonial literatures" is the term that Gefen uses to examine the intersection between literature and care, attesting to how the literary is attempting to construct memory ("faire mémoire"), to make voices heard (2018, 162), thereby underscoring how literary expressions can act as a space from which to redeploy caregiving. This notion of literature's caregiving potential was further explored in the context of a colloquium organized at Sorbonne Université in October 2021 by French scholars Alexandre Gefen and Sandra Laugier and Canada-based scholar Andrea Oberhuber, where the participants (including myself) took up the task of elucidating the relations between literature and caring practices. That is, what are the meaning and expressions of caregiving that take shape in and through literature? How can literature redress the damage and attend to the missing voices? Although we can observe, for example, through the work of scholar Marjorie Deschênes an attempt to detail what "la littérature *care*" (caring literature) is from thematic (explicit portrayal of care and caregivers) and ideological (commitment to social justice, diversity and inclusion of marginalized voices) perspectives, in *Decolonial Care* I am interested in the less overt or self-evident expressions of caregiving in texts.[11] I propose that the articulation of decolonized kinds of care from spaces and contexts where the denial of care is prevalent demands this sense of hesitancy and indefinability. And perhaps quite notably for the purpose of my study by the conclusion of the Paris colloquium on 'caring literature,' the scholarly effort to define the genre remains conspicuously open-ended and incomplete.

MY COMMITMENT TO TEXTUAL PLURALITY AND MULTIDIMENSIONAL CARE

Of course, considering the texts comprising this book, I engage in dialog with scholars such as Marjorie Deschênes, Alexandre Gefen, Andrea Oberhuber, and Sandra Laugier in their exploration of the literary aspects of caregiving. But I have also wanted to reflect a form of textual plurality beyond the limits of prose fiction, adopting an expansive and inclusive understanding of texts and narratives. If, according to French literary critic

Roland Barthes, "text does not stop at (good) Literature," if "it cannot be contained in a hierarchy, even in a simple division of genres," if finally "text always tries to place itself very exactly *behind* the limits of the *doxa*" (1977, 157–158, emphases in original), then throughout *Decolonial Care* I am interested in texts that construct spaces through which to explore the ambivalent nature of caregiving in colonial and neocolonial contexts.

Through this collection of texts lies also the opportunity to recenter the impact of uncaring in the French Caribbean, shedding light on the lives and habitats burdened by the relentless demand for care, as well as to discern practices of care that challenge this historical legacy. This implies that my corpus reflects a reading practice that tends to the many ways through which both caring and uncaring can materialize textually, including specifically close readings of novels and graphic narratives and the interpretation of curatorial work. This approach does not overlook the unique characteristics of each narrative genre and their corresponding analytical terminology. Instead, it involves examining how each text and each context attempt to convey care. It is also imperative to acknowledge, within this study, that these attempts at caregiving are neither uniformly successful nor straightforward. For indeed, they all wrestle with the persistent legacy of colonialism and slavery on the formation of practices of care.

In *Decolonial Care*, I thus emphasize the wide-ranging textual and graphic means by which we can interrogate and elucidate imaginaries of caregiving within the context of the French Caribbean. For example, as regards the comic form with which I, in part, engage in this book, *bande dessinée* artist Jessica Oublié illuminates what she sees as one of the medium's greatest strengths: its capacity to "resist shadows, chronic oblivion, unilateral thinking, competing memories, and a universalism that obfuscates individual and local realities."[12] This assessment of the comic form echoes Oberhuber and Gefen's invitation to "considérer la littérature comme une forme d'action, réparatrice ou transformative" (consider literature as a form of action, restorative or transformative) (2022, §8). When viewed through the lens of care, the texts I include in this study are examined for their textual and graphic strategies to (re)deploy attention, tending to "'voix différentes,' par exemple [celles] de sujets subalternes ou de groupes historiquement minorisés que l'on entend effectivement moins dans nos sociétés dites démocratiques" ("different voices," for example, [those of] subaltern subjects or historically minoritized groups that we actually hear less in our so-called democratic societies) (Oberhuber and Gefen 2022, §4).

Furthermore, my commitment to textual plurality resonates within the multidimensionality of care, which manifests itself across various contexts and in diverse ways. Recalling Tronto and Fisher's definition, which encompasses "everything that we do to maintain, continue, and repair our 'world' so we can live in it as well as possible," one might find the term's definition to be excessively capacious. Therefore, scholars like Silvia Federici (1975) or Arlie Hochschild (2014), particularly in the latter's discussion of "care chains," have insisted instead on caring as labor. This perspective encompasses the day-to-day tasks carried out within the household or as part of the care industry, which are predominantly undertaken by women and often go unpaid or are undervalued. The emphasis on revalorizing care work, endorsed for instance by Federici and Hochschild in their support for reorganizing labor–power relations, adds a layer of specificity to Tronto and Fisher's definition.

In more recent years, theorists in care studies have turned their attention to the ways in which care activities are deployed both in the sphere of human relations and in that of relations between humans and nonhumans; making visible the practices where it is generally women who not only take care of others but also of the environment, thereby highlighting the inequitable environmental burden women tend to experience globally (Hache 2016; Molinier, Laugier, and Falquet 2015). More specifically, concerning care ethics, amid the frenzied exploitation of natural resources and environmental degradation, theorists such as those who contributed to *Genre et environnement: Nouvelles menaces, nouvelles analyses au Nord et au Sud* (Pascale, Laugier, and Falquet 2015), view the environmental crisis as a rich opportunity for reinventing, redeploying, and revaluing care activities. As such, care as method is clearly versatile, intersectional, but also dangerously ubiquitous; for, as Brugère notes, "Alors que le soin concerne une grande partie de notre vie de tous les jours, nous n'en reconnaissons pas la valeur et ne donnons pas à cette dimension l'attention qu'elle mérite" (Although care concerns a large part of our everyday lives, we do not recognize its value and do not give this dimension the attention it deserves) ([2011] 2017, 76). In *Decolonial Care*, I consider four key contexts that, I contend, bring into focus the intersection of care and colonialism: care-focused gender roles; domestic service; nurturing human, in particular women's lives, and environments; and curation as caring. As they are addressed through texts, all these contexts allow for the investigation of the colonial foundations of the ways in which caring has been distributed and uncaring practiced in the islands of Guadeloupe and Martinique, while also enabling the conceptualization of a decolonial care from and for the Caribbean region.

METHODOLOGY: CONSIDERING THE DECOLONIZATION OF CARE THROUGH THE DUAL AXIS OF CARING AND UNCARING

Whatever the focus of care—toward people in historical and contemporary contexts (care-focused gender roles, domestic service, and curation) or the environment (informed by ecofeminist thought)—*Decolonial Care* engages its ambivalent nature. In the different settings in which attitudes of care become manifest, this book addresses the effect of the more or less overt "I don't care" dispositions from past and present times. For indeed, *Decolonial Care* argues that to imagine caregiving in the context of the French Caribbean means reckoning with intrinsically uncaring practices inherited from colonial rule that show disregard for human life and environments. As such, putting in dialogue postcolonial studies and care studies, this book first aims to elucidate how caring and uncaring have been historically shaped by colonialism.

Second, *Decolonial Care* questions how we can emerge from diverse and overlapping forms of uncaring. As such, the reflection on care throughout this book is situated in the knowing, in recognition of the conceptual challenges posed by the (neo)colonial systemic neglect inherent in historical asymmetrical demands for care. Navigating the underexplored intersection of care and colonialism, this study thus underscores the complexities of reimagining caregiving through a decolonial lens within contemporary landscapes that are still very much shaped by (neo)colonial power dynamics and exploitation.

I take as my point of departure eight primary texts, encompassing both visual and textual forms: the curatorial discourse behind the Paris exhibition *Black Models, from Géricault to Matisse* (March 26–July 21, 2019); Fabienne Kanor's novel *Humus* (2006); Gisèle Pineau's novel *Morne Câpresse* (2008), Jessica Oublié et al. graphic narrative *Tropiques toxiques* (2020), Françoise Ega's memoir *Lettres à une Noire* (1978), Jessica Oublié and Marie-Ange Rousseau's graphic narrative *Péyi an nou* (2017), Kanor's novel *D'eaux douces* (2004), and Gaël Octavia's novel *La bonne histoire de Madeleine Démétrius* (2020) (in the order they are studied in this book). I read for what I call the dual axis of caring and uncaring. This approach emphasizes the inseparability of care from its obscured counterpart, uncaring. Each chapter thus in turn reflects this inherent ambivalence. By traversing this dual axis, I consider the complexities surrounding the decolonization of care. This entails documenting the damaging impact of colonialism and slavery on practices of care while also contributing to the development of decolonial approaches to care that sustain human life and livable environments in French Caribbean contexts.

Chapter Organization

CHAPTER 1: CURATING SILENCES

Confronting the erasure of personal narratives and identities in the context of slavery and colonization, chapter 1 explores the ways in which the lives of previously silenced individuals are portrayed in postcolonial contexts. In doing so, this chapter interrogates attempts to repair the damage caused by dehumanizing practices in the economic, ideological, and epistemic spheres.

This chapter first examines the limits of restoring the lost names of individuals who served as models in well-known works of art. I focus on the exhibition *Le modèle noir, de Géricault à Matisse* (Black models: from Géricault to Matisse), which took place at the Musée d'Orsay in Paris between March 26 and July 21, 2019, and I consider, to a lesser extent, its iteration at the Mémorial ACTe in Guadeloupe, under the title *Le modèle noir, de Géricault à Picasso* (Black models: from Géricault to Picasso, September 14 to December 29, 2019). The curators of this traveling exhibition attempted to recover the names of Black models in order to rehumanize them. However, this chapter argues that, when the curators failed in their attempt to retrieve all the names of the individuals depicted in the artwork, they engaged in conjecture and devised problematic new names for individuals and some works of art. This inauthentic way of reconstructing the historical narrative isolates the works from the cultural contexts in which they were produced. The study of the *Modèle noir* exhibition ultimately serves as an example of a failed attempt at caring because it covers up the erasure, rather than repairing it or even simply acknowledging it.

I place this example of caring gone wrong in contrast with an analysis of Fabienne Kanor's novel *Humus* (2006), arguing that the recognition of what has been lost and fractured by the legacy of colonialism is essential to an effective practice of care. Kanor uses her novel to underscore how historical accounts of the lives of the enslaved are scarce, incomplete, and objectifying. Kanor prefaces

Humus by telling the story of her visit to the departmental archives of the city of Nantes in France where she learned of an incident that took place in 1774 aboard a slave ship: fourteen unnamed African women escaped the ship's hold and leapt overboard all at once to resist their enslavement. Only six of them survived while the others drowned or were killed by sharks. "How to tell, how to retell this story told by men?" (9), Kanor asks. How, indeed? Motivated by "a desire to swap [or] to trade away technical discourse for the spoken word," Kanor's novel tells fictionalized versions of the experience of each of these women (Humus 2020). All the while, rather than provide cohesive narratives for each of these women, the author retains important aspects of the original erasure, restituting the violence of this oppression through truncated sentences and fragments of memory.

This chapter, then, opens the book by exploring the tension between our responsibility in reckoning with gaps in the historical records and the act of repairing and caregiving. Inhabiting this tension allows us to engage with the complexity of France's colonial legacy in the Atlantic world by responsibly giving voice to previously marginalized lives and experiences.

CHAPTER 2: VOICES OF THE BUMIDOM, OR THE COLONIAL LEGACY OF CARE WORK

The second chapter examines care work from the perspective of the BUMIDOM, in particular the institutionalization of domesticity in migration from the French Caribbean to hexagonal France. The BUMIDOM was a government-led agency aimed at organizing migration primarily from the French Caribbean (Guadeloupe and Martinique) and Réunion between the years 1963 and 1982. Over the course of its existence, the BUMIDOM supervised a total of 186,289 departures, including 63,505 migrants from Guadeloupe, 43,516 from Martinique, and 76,583 from Réunion. As part of this controlled migration, low-paid jobs dominated, and departmental migration was distributed in specific sectors of the French economy. This chapter explores the intersection of caregiving and the history of the BUMIDOM, which has been largely shrouded in silence, as well as investigates ways to attend to the voices that have been historically dismissed or self-repressed.

An analysis of Ega's 1978 epistolary memoir *Lettres à une Noire* in the first part of this chapter helps analyze the organization of care work as part of the BUMIDOM, especially the colonial continuities in the distribution of care work that prolonged inequalities between hexagonal France and its overseas departments on the basis of class, gender, and race. Ega's personal account of the BUMIDOM years not only refuses the silence around the BUMIDOM but more importantly develops kinds of attention that disrupt a hierarchy of attention that favors those who disproportionately demand care, to focus instead on the experiences of caregivers.

In keeping with an emphasis on shifting forms of attention, the second half of this chapter provides an analysis of *Péyi an nou* (Kreyòl for "our country", 2017), a graphic narrative by Jessica Oublié (scenarist) and Marie-Ange Rousseau (illustrator) that gives us further insight into the quiet memories of the BUMIDOM, making them emerge in the present day. Through an emphasis on the interplay between BUMIDOM and care, this chapter places care work within the history of colonialism and slavery and its legacy while also analyzing the formal expressions in literary and graphic texts that emphasize voices of the BUMIDOM.

CHAPTER 3: INHABITING THE LAND AFTER ENVIRONMENTAL DAMAGE

Chapter 3 shifts attention to the impact of blatant uncaring practices toward people and the environment resulting from colonial extractivism and exploitation of the land in the French Antilles. The literary representations of a damaged Caribbean landscape and habitat—"your home, the place you are from" (Kincaid 2020)—very much underscore the effects of uncaring while also contributing to the formation of caring experimental futures. In this chapter, I am particularly interested in looking at depictions of the Caribbean landscape as a site dramatically altered by "colonial inhabitation" (Ferdinand 2019), as well as the ways in which we can reimagine human interaction with that landscape. How does the literary negotiate the tension between the inescapability of colonial damage and the possibility of recovery? I explore two ways of responding to colonial appropriation, exploitation, and extraction.

First, in *Morne Câpresse* by Gisèle Pineau (2008) we see a community of women cloister themselves away from the violence they have endured as well as from a habitat ravaged by (neo)colonial practices. The Congrégation des Filles de Cham (the Congregation of the Daughters of Cham) is an independent community attempting to subsist, through gardening and solidarity, away from the devastated "monde d'en-bas" (world below). Imagined as the site that would repair socioeconomic distress, the congregation is first modeled as a *locus amoenus*, transforming a former plantation into an enclosed garden space. Despite this effort to newly cultivate the land, this aspiring sanctuary covers up the history of the plantation while also silencing the women it intends to heal.

Second, in *Tropiques toxiques* (Toxic tropics, 2020) by Jessica Oublié et al., readers are introduced to the ways in which those who remain on the damaged land attempt to cope with and adapt to a new postcolonial reality. Oublié's investigative work highly contributes to the knowledge on chlordecone, a toxic pesticide used in banana plantations to eradicate weevils between the years 1972 and 1993 in Guadeloupe and Martinique. The graphic narrative sheds light on the harmful effect of chlordecone exposure on food and water sustainability as well as on traditional lifestyles, such as the Creole garden. In contrast to the escapism of *Morne Câpresse*, *Tropiques toxiques* grapples with the lasting effect of toxicity on people and lived environments. The graphic narrative foregrounds local and individual attempts to compensate for the French government's inaction with respect to widespread chlordecone contamination.

Once explored alongside each other, these two narratives reveal the impossibility of escape from the past and the need to develop solutions in light of the environmental and human legacies of colonialism. I argue that these texts, therefore, contain a proposition for expansive and lucid caring imaginaries: expansive in the sense that they consider the human and nonhuman worlds in their interconnectedness and lucid in the sense that they recognize continuity with the past. This chapter frames these contrasting literary imaginaries as a template to inhabit the "world below" and resist the legacy of colonial environmental violence.

CHAPTER 4: REBELLIOUS CARE, OR DECONSTRUCTING THE MYTH OF THE *POTO-MITAN* WOMAN

A crucial goal of care studies is to challenge the assumption that care is primarily a woman's responsibility, emphasizing instead the importance of care as a human value and political ideal. This chapter starts by questioning the assignment of women to care through the figure of the *poto-mitan* woman (*fanm potomitan* in Kreyòl). Poto-mitan traditionally refers to the central pillar of Haitian vodou temples, a pillar that supports the building's entire weight. By way of metaphor, the term also applies in Antillean cultures to the "mère-courage" (courageous mother), the strong "wife-mother" who holds together the household, hiding any sign of emotional distress and simultaneously relieving responsibility from male figures.

Through the analysis of Fabienne Kanor's novel *D'eaux douces* (Fresh waters, 2004), I start by exploring a refusal of the relegation to care, introducing the concept of rebellious care. In Kanor's novel, the main protagonist, Frida, interrogates a cycle of self-resignation that she inherited from her mother, who encouraged her from childhood to be self-reliant, self-effacing, and nurturing in relation to men. Eventually, Frida violently breaks the cycle by murdering her lover, Eric, and killing herself. In analyzing Frida's actions in the light of rebellious care, this chapter argues that *D'eaux douces* shows both the limits of a destructive cycle passed on through the generations as well as the necessity to imagine a path away from the constraints of a pressing responsibility to care for women.

I then juxtapose the example of rebellious care in Kanor's novel with Gaël Octavia's novel *La bonne histoire de Madeleine Démétrius* (Madeleine Démétrius's good story, 2020) in order to explore emancipation from the figure of the *poto-mitan* woman. Indeed, Octavia's novel opens with an encounter between the narrator, a writer who left Martinique to settle in hexagonal France, and her long-lost high school friend, Madeleine Démétrius. Démétrius entrusts her friend with a troubling story from their childhood. Through a dive into the past, the narrative peels away the layers of fictionalization of the *poto-mitan* woman across generations to expose the concept's fallacy, as well as lay bare its profound impact on the distribution of caregiving responsibilities.

This chapter argues that while Kanor's novel shows the bankruptcy of the *poto-mitan* as a figure, Octavia's novel supports competing representations of women in their relations to each other, to male figures, and to those who come after them.

CODA: GISÈLE PINEAU, OR THE LITERARY VOICE OF A CAREGIVER

This book's conclusion proposes an analysis of *Folie, aller simple: Journée ordinaire d'une infirmière* (Madness, a one-way ticket: an ordinary day in the life of a nurse, 2010) by Gisèle Pineau, in which the author recounts her work as a psychiatric nurse. After working for thirty years in a psychiatric hospital in Guadeloupe, Pineau moved to the Paris region where she continued to practice nursing. This autobiographical text describes a typical day in a psychiatric hospital, in particular nurses' interactions with mentally ill patients and Pineau's reflections on her activity as a caregiver and on her role as a writer.

Taking an interest in these two activities performed in parallel, the book's coda explores formal links between providing care (as a nurse) and writing as a caring activity, both for the self as well as for those who give or receive care. As Pineau writes about the lives of those pushed to the margins, this text allows me to explore writing about caregiving as well as literature as a means of deploying fundamental gestures of care, such as attentiveness, responsibility, and responsiveness. I argue that these gestures are not limited to the health care workforce; they are relevant to other socioeconomic, professional, and artistic spheres.

An Ethic of Care in Scholarly and Analytical Practices

Throughout *Decolonial Care*, I propose that reading for decolonial interpretations of caregiving within the intersectional framework of care studies and French Caribbean studies can serve as a means to develop attention to texts that actively take on the question of care. The texts comprising my corpus, whether graphic or not, grapple with ways to elucidate and build imaginaries of caregiving, thereby amplifying the textuality of care. These texts express, each in their own way, the refusal of a legacy of carelessness, ultimately seeking to transform the ways care manifests across story worlds.

Drawing inspiration from scholars such as Christina Sharpe (*In the Wake: On Blackness and Being*, 2016), Régine Michelle Jean-Charles deploys an "ethic of care" in her study *Looking for Other Worlds: Black Feminism and Haitian Fiction* (2022). For Jean-Charles, this ethic entails "engaging a practice of deep reading inviting us readers and scholars to pay attention to the messages embedded in the narratives for the characters and for ourselves as well as the embodied principles of Black feminist thought" (7). Reading with care, therefore, suggests being guided by the prospect of uncovering alternative worlds and subsequently questioning and reconfiguring our own lived experiences anew. In this sense, as readers, we can remain receptive to the possibilities that might emerge from texts and resonate with what Jean-Charles terms "our own ethical imaginations" (10).

Here, truly, care concerns not only the revelations about care that texts may contain, but also the meditative scholarly and readerly practice that questions the mechanics of textual and graphical landscapes to illuminate how care has been informed by the history of colonialism and slavery and how imaginaries of caregiving become manifest in French Caribbean contexts beyond or despite this legacy. However, as we have seen and will continue to see the task of decolonizing care is confronted with the persistence of uncaring. As such, this task is not self-evident; it requires work and is susceptible to deviate from its intended course. But, for now, let us dare to care.

1
Curating Silences

The transatlantic slave trade constitutes a devastating abyss. Through the Middle Passage, the sea has become witness to the loss of subjecthood of millions of deported Africans, a site of historical dispossession as well as physical and figurative death. For Martinican thinker Édouard Glissant, the abyss (*gouffre* in French) represents precisely the destructive experience of deportation from Africa to the Americas.[1] The triple abyss conceptualized by Glissant—the hold of the slave ship ("le ventre de la barque"), the sea ("l'abîme marin"), and everything that has been left behind ("tout cela qui a été abandonné") or the Former Land ("le Pays d'Avant")—is not only useful to interpret the experience of displacement but also to account for the dispersed, unclaimed, and severed biographical threads through the making of African captives into human commodities. "We declare slaves to be charges, and as such enter into community property": article XLIV is found, alongside fifty-nine other articles, in the *Code Noir* enacted by King Louis XIV in 1685 to define the legal status of the enslaved in the French colonial empire. To be enslaved, then, meant to be assigned monetary value, to be subsumed into a knowledge system where the enslaved are viewed in terms of calculability and profit. Within "an economic system in which race demarcated human beings as property," the condition of slavery stabilized a racial hierarchy, a system of classification that denied deported Africans their individuality and freedom (Morgan 2021, 4).

In European visual culture of the late eighteenth century, one of the most familiar images of the slave ship is the depiction of enslaved Africans chained together in the hold below decks, in "rows of Black bodies laid out like sardines in a can" to borrow from the description by art historian David Bindman in *The Black Figure in the European Imaginary* (2017, 11).[2] The image, created in 1787, is a diagram of the *Brookes* of Liverpool, titled "Description of a Slave Ship." Although the print was instrumental in campaigning for the abolition of the slave trade (mainly across Great Britain at the time), it also inaugurated a troubling visuality for Black bodies as part of the European imaginary.[3] The diagram shows the captives, hardly distinguishable from one another, shackled together and forced to remain lying down side by side for the most part of the voyage; bodies are arranged so as to maximize space, amassed so as to anticipate the death of the enslaved during the transatlantic journey. Ship crowding, then, illuminates the intersection of the economic rationality informing the transportation methods of enslaved people and the dispossession and dehumanization of Black bodies within European ideological thought.

Considering Africans were present in Europe "since Roman times at least," I find the ideological rationalization that undergirds the creation of commodified Black bodies as part of the slave system reflected in European visual arts—not limited to slave ship diagrams (Bindman 2017, 12). Africans present in Europe in the seventeenth century "had come as slaves, singled out from the masses abducted from Africa for roles in wealthy households as personal servants, footmen, horse grooms, or, in the case of small children, pets for the ladies of the court or the household" (12). The conditions of their presence under the racialized category of the enslaved, or the colonized, often rendered them absent from historical accounts of individual lives. Confronting the crushing reality of historically obscured lives, this chapter explores the ways in which the silenced individualities of the enslaved and colonized are represented and reckoned with in postcolonial contexts, asking what it means to repair, if at all possible, the damage caused by ideological, historical, and epistemic forms of erasure. This chapter delves into the complexities of effective caregiving in addressing the erasure of the enslaveds' past, examining two distinct types of text: Fabienne Kanor's novel *Humus* and the curatorial discourses surrounding the exhibition *Le modèle noir, de Géricault à Matisse* (Black models: from Géricault to Matisse) at the Musée d'Orsay in Paris from March 26 to July 21, 2019, and to a lesser extent its iteration at the Mémorial ACTe in Guadeloupe, where it was titled *Le modèle noir, de Géricault à Picasso* (Black models, from Géricault to Picasso) from September 14 to December 29, 2019.[4] By analyzing these texts, this chapter will illuminate the limits of purported forms of care made manifest in the curatorial discourses surrounding the "Black Models" exhibitions while also investigating Kanor's strategies in *Humus* to confront the historical dispossession and invisibilization of the enslaved and colonized within the broader context of the Black Atlantic.

In theories of care, as early as in the 1980s there has been a clear focus on what "the values of caring—attentiveness, responsibility, nurturance, compassion, nurturing others' needs"—can achieve to make visible and to listen attentively to the invisibilized, the "relatively disenfranchised in the political world," the individuals whose voices are often devalued and not heard (Tronto 1993, 3, 21). But what kind of care can be imagined for the lives and the voices that disappeared without a trace, "lost to the pages of legislative debates, merchant ledgers, and calculations of risk, finance, fluctuating value, tariffs, products, and trade" (Morgan 2021, 9)? As historian Jennifer L. Morgan has noted, commenting on the portrait on the cover of her book (*Portrait of an African Woman Holding a Clock*, 1583, by Annibale Carracci), "at the time when the woman was painted, the legality of African enslavability had circulated around the Mediterranean for almost 150 years—but art historians don't know who this woman is. They can't" (2021, ix). For indeed, the damage caused by slavery and colonialism cannot be reversed, rendering the task of narrating silenced lives initially daunting, if not seemingly impossible.

Echoing the words of scholar Saidiya Hartman as she grapples with the challenges of recounting the story of Venus, the emblematic figure of the enslaved woman, in her essay "Venus in Two Acts" (2008), we ponder, "How does one recuperate lives entangled with and impossible to differentiate from the terrible utterances that condemned them to death?" (3). As we grapple with the initial impossibility of narrating silenced lives, I propose directing our focus toward the knowledge systems that produced the erasure of voice. It is through this process of acknowledging the lasting impact of erasure, loss, and death that I suggest we may locate the potential for caregiving.

Gisèle Pineau's 2007 memoir *Mes quatre femmes* gives a compelling account of the tension between discontinued or lost personal narratives and the urge to preserve the voices of four of her ancestors: Angélique, who was born enslaved in Guadeloupe in 1792; the two sisters Gisèle and Daisy; and Julia, Daisy's mother-in-law and grandmother of the narrator (Pineau). Pineau describes a difficult but forced negotiation with inherited absence:

> Se contenter de cet unique cliché. Faire son deuil des reliques qui n'ont pas subsisté. Se fabriquer une histoire avec si peu de pistes. Se revêtir de ce prénom chagrin. Inquiète, l'endosser tel un habit prêté. (57–58)

> You have to accept a single photograph. You have to mourn relics that have ceased to exist. You have to fabricate a history with very few traces. And to take on this *prénom chagrin*. Anxiously, you have to adopt it like a borrowed garment.

In the absence of birth certificates or certified documents, the four women in Pineau's memoir acknowledge a wounded personal and family history that they are empowered to reclaim, question, and eventually redeem as they come together within the fictional space. Here, by focusing on voices and experiences that have long been neglected, Pineau identifies the practice of care (perhaps also self-care) as rooted in acknowledging an irreparable loss; this is a necessary step for Pineau to have a liberated relationship with her past and envision the future. More broadly, attempts to engage with what has been lost manifest in diverse forms, prompting us to consider what defines caring practices amid the various approaches to the invisibilized and fragmented lives of the enslaved and colonized. I am thus interested in interrogating the acts of curation that engage through texts with the absences produced by slavery and colonialism. Through this exploration, I contend that the recognition of what has been lost and fractured by the legacy of colonialism and slavery is essential to decolonial practices of care in the present.

As I initiate my exploration of the diverse methodologies for curating historical silences through texts, I wish to underscore the particular significance of the *Modèle noir* exhibition. Numerous exhibitions have been created in France in recent years seeking to be witness to the French colonial and slave past. These include the exhibition *L'Abîme: Nantes dans la traite atlantique et l'esclavage colonial, 1707–1830*, which took place at the Château des Ducs de Bretagne: Musée d'Histoire de Nantes, from October 16, 2021, to June 19, 2022, and the exhibition *Marronnage: L'art de briser ses chaines*, which took place at the Maison d'Amérique Latine in Paris from May 12, 2022, to September 24, 2022.[5] However, the Musée d'Orsay's *Modèle noir* exhibition was the first to propose an *exclusive* focus on the portrayal of Black individuals in French art, from the end of the eighteenth century to the mid-twentieth century. This exhibition marked a groundbreaking effort at redressing the silences surrounding the lives of Black individuals within the context of slavery and colonialism; it was, as French historian Laurent Martin justly notes, "la première fois qu'un grand musée français montait une telle exposition, qui vient à son heure dans un pays qui s'interroge de plus en plus sur la place faite, dans les arts, les médias, la société dans son ensemble, aux minorités visibles—ou invisible" (the first time that a major French museum has created such an exhibition, which comes at the right time in a country that is increasingly questioning the place given in the arts, the media, and society as a whole to visible—or invisible— minorities) (235).

Regarding my approach to curation, while initially informed by an analysis of the *Modèle noir* exhibitions, I wish to already signal that it will not be limited to museum curatorial practice and later a study of Kanor's novel *Humus*. In point of fact, the term invites a broader reflection on practices of care. The substantive *curation* quite fittingly takes on a double meaning: one refers to the organization and maintaining of an art exhibition, a museum, or a gallery; the other resonates with the Latin roots of the word— *curatio*, past participle of *curo* or *curare*, which means "to take care of," especially in the sense of curing, restoring to health. The act of restoring, of reclaiming the biographies of silenced models in colonial Paris seems in fact central to the curatorial team formed by Cécile Debray, Stéphane Guégan, Denise Murrell, and Isolde Pludermacher (2019). The introduction to the exhibition catalog provides the means to elucidate at least in part their curatorial intention:

> Un prénom ou un surnom a longtemps suffi, au mieux, à les [ces protagonistes oubliés de l'histoire de l'art] désigner. Le nom est la première chose que les esclaves se font voler, a dit Césaire. L'une de nos ambitions prioritaires fut d'emblée de retrouver l'identité de modèles d'atelier longtemps restés anonymes, et de mettre en évidence leur histoire et leur parcours. L'enquête, la reconquête d'une histoire souvent caricaturée, commençait là. (15)

> A name or a surname has for a long time been enough, in the best of circumstances, to identify those forgotten protagonists of art history. Their name is the first thing that was stolen from slaves, Césaire said. One of our main priorities was to

immediately retrieve the identity of the studio models who had long remained anonymous and to underscore their story and experience. The investigation, the reclaiming of a history often caricatured, was starting there.

Inspired by the work of Denise Murrell (2014) undertaken in part to lift the prevailing silence surrounding the real-life story of Laure, the Black maid in Édouard Manet's 1863 painting *Olympia*, among other models, the curators adopted a restorative practice. First, they adapted the titles of artworks to our contemporary present by replacing racially marked terms with a more neutral—that is, less offensive—wording. Second, they renamed, if possible, Black models who had been until now unknown.[6]

For instance, a sketch by French painter and printmaker Henri Guérard originally was titled *Une Négresse, d'après Eva Gonzalès*. The new name, *Jeune femme de profil* (Laure?), *d'après Eva Gonzalès* (emphasis mine), encapsulates the two kinds of restorative strategies endorsed by the curators of the *Modèle noir* exhibition. First, "une négresse" becomes "jeune femme," privileging the ascription of gender and age over a derogatory racialized term, for obvious reasons. Second, Laure, the Black model who posed for Manet's *Olympia*, may or may not be the model for Guérard's sketch; an unresolved uncertainty, contained in the question mark placed immediately after what is no more than a guess, remains. When, then, does the act of restoring individuality risk producing another effacement of the specific conditions of existence that have historically been under erasure? What are the limits of a revisionary narrative when there is an existing tension with the ideological and colonial processes that produced erasure at the time? Belief in the restorative potential of the act of renaming, even if partial, may help sustain caring relations between more or less distant others in our contemporary present while also inaugurating a culture and politics of inclusion for the future. However, the ways we choose to tell the past engage our present relationship to that same past, revealing an active acknowledgment of the history and legacy of colonialism—or an unwitting replaying thereof.

France's colonial past and the lasting impact of slavery and colonialism are still largely underdiscussed or are awkwardly mitigated in contemporary French political and social life. For example, on February 23, 2005, a law regarding teaching about colonial history was passed by the National Assembly (repealed in 2006 by President Jacques Chirac [1995–2007]) to require high school teachers to teach the "positive values" of colonialism. More recently, on January 3, 2022, Valerie Pecresse, the right-wing LR (Les Républicains) presidential candidate, denied that slavery and colonialism constituted crimes against humanity (in the same way as the Shoah, which was her counterexample); she defended the mythical (male) "heroes" of the French nation and the *bonnes choses* ("good aspects") of colonization. It seems premature, to say the least, to sideline too promptly the ideology and economy of racial classification and hierarchy that formed the crux of colonialism and slavery as relics of the past. As Haitian anthropologist Michel-Rolph Trouillot has noted, "to condemn slavery alone is the easy way out" (1995, 148); for indeed, there is a danger in singling out the past in a fixed and self-enclosed social system.

Numerous models represented in artworks of the late nineteenth century (on display at the 2019 exhibition) settled in Paris after the second abolition of slavery in 1848, but the construction of human hierarchies, racialized categories of difference, and technologies of erasure (such as the numerical values of human lives) had already impregnated social relations and French society at large.[7] We can agree that terms such as *câpresse*, *mulâtresse*, and *négresse*, once part of common speech, cannot be used today, in a way similar to the curators' plea in the introductory panel to the exhibition.[8] But considering the blind spots, omissions, and denials in France's reckoning with its colonial past, to simply rename the Black models in French art history extracts them from a past world, that of colonial Paris, and reinscribes them in a "separate world" (to use Trouillot's terminology), an aspiring-to-be-caring world. However, this a priori restorative attitude glances over the production of these nameless others (in this case, the Black models) in the past as well as over the lasting effects of such an externally constructed ideological model on so-perceived individuals.

Quite distinctively, as part of the Guadeloupean iteration of the *Modèle noir* exhibit, a pedagogical dossier was produced, including a proposition by French teacher of history and geography and project manager in the educational service of the Fabre Museum in Montpellier, Vivien Chabanne, to organize a debate on the decision to rename artworks that contain racist terminology (Deriau-Reine and Louzon-Gamba 2019, 46–63). Using the example of French painter Frédéric Bazille's *Jeune femme aux pivoines* (1870; formerly titled *La négresse aux pivoines*), which was renamed in the context of the "Adjustment of Colonial Terminology" program at the Rijksmuseum in Amsterdam, the dossier invites instructors and students to reflect on the ethical implications of the removal of racially charged terms, considering the potential effacement of colonial and racist history.[9] The debate is organized around two central questions: (1) "Faut-il mettre fin à une terminologie discriminatoire pour ne pas offenser des personnes qui se sentiraient blessées par ces mots?" (Should we put an end to discriminatory terminology so as to not offend people who would feel hurt by these words?); and (2) "Faut-il au contraire la conserver comme le témoignage d'un contexte historique?" (On the contrary, should it be preserved as the testimony of a historical context?). Chabanne clarifies that the goal is not to "faire un choix entre le bien et le mal" (make a choice between good and evil) but rather to become aware of and participate in an ongoing questioning amid museum collections with regard to curation of artworks that reflect colonial imaginaries. Through this, the Guadeloupean edition of the *Modèle noir* exhibition acknowledges, at least in its paratext, the potential for debate surrounding curatorial strategies that navigate the complex interplay between embracing expressions of individuality and confronting colonial practices of collective erasure.

Of course, the restorative practice that seeks to develop attention to the individual, the particular, is in some respects commendable and has clearly been advocated for by many in recent years. We have seen the expansion of biographical projects about the African and Caribbean presence during the colonial period with works such as historian Robin Mitchell's *Vénus Noire* (2020) or Congolese writer Bona Mangangu's *Joseph Le Maure* (2016). It is, however, crucial to pay special attention to the present within which the act of repairing is being conducted and to consider who, why, and how. For example, Mangangu's text seeks to give a voice to Joseph, born in the French colony of Saint-Domingue (present day Haiti) circa 1793, who was hired as a regular model for the École des Beaux-Arts in 1832 and is especially known for working with Théodore Géricault. Mangangu wants to create intimacy between the two men as Joseph is on a first-name basis with Théodore. But what Mangangu eventually delivers is a glorifying portrayal of Géricault: "Théodore s'est dressé contre les tenants de l'Unique. Il est mort, animé par la volonté farouche de comprendre la vérité de l'autre, la rose du songe serrée dans son jeune cœur de trente et deux printemps" (Theodore rose against the defenders of the Unique. He died, moved by the fierce desire to understand the truth of the Other, holding the rose of dreams against his heart at the young age of thirty-two). This may be a genuine appreciation of the painter's work, but it still fails to displace the focus from the long-celebrated *Maître*.

With Mangangu's somewhat shaky unveiling of Joseph's personal history, the possible limitations of the act of renaming alone appear all the more visible. Put differently, Mangangu's narrative is undoubtedly limited by a crushing threefold production of anonymity at the time when Joseph lived, related to framings of, first, the growing working classes; second, of the care workers as part of this working class, and finally, of the Black presence in nineteenth-century Europe. We see in an industrializing Europe by the middle of the nineteenth century the increasing numbers of workers moving to and settling in urban centers, the *sans-part* to borrow an expression from French philosopher Jacques Rancière (1992). According to Rancière, figures of the poor throughout history, such as the plebs in Antiquity, the Third Estate, or the industrial proletariat, are commonly identified as an anonymized supernumerary social group, reduced to hard-working bodies. In the nineteenth century, artists' models, except in the case of commissioned portraits mostly by members of the aristocracy and bourgeoisie, were hourly workers hired as part of a "temporary commercial exchange," as art historian Susan Waller explains in her study *The Invention of the Model* ([2006] 2017). As part of this economy of bodies, Waller identifies a shift in the artist–model transaction, noting that, unlike in the eighteenth century, "models were no longer an integral part of the institution [the Académie des Beaux-Arts, later known as the École des Beaux-Arts]: while "the two *modèles à l'année* continued to be paid 550 francs per year," the occasional models were "hired by the pose" and "paid 60 francs for a two-week period" (18).[10]

The encounter between artists and models, then, becomes profoundly shaped by precarious labor conditions. For indeed, while the working class was becoming a prominent subject of art in nineteenth-century European visual arts, professional or occasional *poseurs·ses* inherently bound to this social group made scarce, often vague if not depreciative, apparitions in official records such as artists' notebooks or correspondence, alphabetical directories, and payslips.[11] For example, the few remaining traces known to this day of the Black maid in Manet's *Olympia* are very limited: they include, as Murrell reminds us, a brief reference to her in one of Manet's notebook entries in late 1862, which reads "Laure, très belle négresse" (Laure, very beautiful Negress) and reveals that Laure "lived at 11 rue Vintimille, just below the Place de Clichy, less than a ten-minute walk from Manet's studio" (9).[12] Such vagueness surrounding models at the time, who were usually recorded under a first name or nickname and very rarely under a family name, gives evidence that the emerging working classes of the nineteenth century were included into a hierarchical distribution of social roles contributing to the invisibilization and categorization of certain types of workers.[13]

When Estelle Bégué and Isolde Pludermacher discuss, in their catalog essay, the diffuse identity of models in nineteenth-century Paris, the two curators adopt a universalizing discourse, perhaps in an attempt to neutralize the possibly unfair treatment of Black workers: "Si la présence de Parisiens noirs au XIXe siècle est rendue visible à travers de nombreuses oeuvres d'art, leur identité demeure le plus souvent une énigme, *mais il convient de rappeler que c'est généralement le cas pour tous les modèles, quelle que soit leur couleur de peau*" (If the presence of Black Parisians in nineteenth century is made visible in numerous works of art, their identity remains in most cases a mystery, *but it is important to not forget that it is usually the case for all models, regardless of their skin color*) (Debray et al. 2019, 196, emphasis mine). In the context of the Guadeloupean edition of the *Modèle noir* exhibition, Martial similarly highlights the constraints of identifying Black individuals represented in European visual arts from the eighteenth to the twentieth century, attributing it broadly to a lack of census ("faute de recensement" in French; Deriau-Reine and Louzon-Gamba 2019, 7). This being said, it might appear clumsy to disqualify in a contemporary context a culture of anonymity that contributed to the prevailing production of social and racial types, an ideological model that has clearly privileged the production of individual types over individuality.

The impulse toward a scopic classifying vision of society at the time is in fact reflected in the genre of "panoramic literature" that German philosopher Walter Benjamin describes in his unfinished and posthumously published *Arcades Project* as "individual sketches" in "anecdotal form" (2003, 6). Examples in literature include the encyclopedic multivolume *Les français peints par eux-mêmes* published by Léon-Henri Curmer between 1840 and 1842 where we find an exposé on, among other "types," the "nourrice sur place" or "on-site nanny" by Amédée Achard that starts on an ominous note:

> Si j'avais l'honneur d'être père de famille, je n'oserais pas écrire cet article, tant je craindrais d'exposer ma race au ressentiment des nourrices futures; il y a trop de qualités, trop de péchés mondains, trop de qualités négatives à dévoiler. La seule chose qui pourrait peut-être accroître mon courage, c'est cette pensée consolante qu'en général les nourrices ne savent pas lire. (1:17)
>
> If I had the honor to be a father, I would not dare write this article, as I would fear to expose my race to the resentment of future nannies; there are too many attributes, too many social sins, too many negative qualities to reveal. The only thing that would increase my courage is the comforting thought that in general nannies cannot read.

This tendency toward classifying and stereotyping the multitudes passing through or residing in nineteenth-century urban centers (mostly Paris) inaugurates the production of controlled social realities reified or made-familiar subsets of the everyday crowd.

Both literary and visual art forms emerge in the panoramic genre as the prime site of representation of prescriptive traits ascribed to social but also racial types in this "century obsessed with representation" (De Margerie and Papet 2004, 127). Among the works displayed at the Parisian exhibition, sculptures by Charles Cordier, such as *Buste de nègre du Soudan* (1857; renamed *Homme du Soudan français*) or *Câpresse* or *Négresse des colonies* (1861; renamed *Femmes des colonies*), resonate with the artist's intention "to create a gallery of busts of the human races" (De Margerie and Papet 2004, 13) at a time when the Other, the allegedly foreign, was rarely represented in European artistic circles.[14] By placing his work at the intersection of the artistic and the ethnographic, Cordier, a member of the Society of Anthropology, can be considered an "artist-ethnographer." As art historian Charmaine Nelson explains in her 2010 study *Representing the Black Female Subject in Western Art*, "traveling to France's North African colonies on a grant of one thousand francs, his task was to portray racial 'types' through the amalgamation of individuals into composites"; moreover, Nelson adds, "works like his *Nègre du Soudan* ou *Nègre en costume algérien* (1856–1857) were intended for the new ethnographic gallery in the Musée national d'Histoire naturelle in Paris" (165).[15] And, in fact, Adrienne Childs and Susan Libby call our attention to the fact that "works were often titled 'Negro,' 'Negress,' and 'Study of a Black,' marking the Blackness of the figure as the central subject" (2017, 23)—that is, the racial type rather than the individual figure. Therefore, while David Bindman makes mention of Cordier's note that "le beau n'est pas propre à une race privilégiée" (beauty does not belong to a single, privileged race) in the exhibition catalog (Debray et al. 2019, 108), the idea that beauty is everywhere should not distract us from the fact that the artist's project partakes in the racialization of the world's peoples, documenting and recording constructed racial types over individuals.

Models, as part of this taxonomy, find themselves acting out classifiable social and racial types. Social and racial typology is complemented by the prevalence of care workers among whom we find a large majority of marginalized social groups, in particular women arriving in hexagonal France from the Caribbean in the second half of the nineteenth century. Care work (in its professionalized form), such as nursing, home health care, the labor of caring for children and other dependents today, has historically been undervalued, underpaid, and dominated by women, migrant workers, and people who identify as belonging to minority groups (Barbagallo and Federici 2012; Brugère 2011; Ibos et al. 2019; Paperman and Laugier 2006; Tronto 1993, 2013).[16] The allocation of caring responsibilities in this context concerns the issue of disempowerment attached to the racial and gender organization of care work and the devaluation of care work more generally. In the arts, Black models were set to represent the most dominant social and racial realities of the time, acting out the maid in Manet's *Olympia* (1863) or the nanny in Jacques-Eugène Feyen's *Le baiser enfantin* (1865). They reveal both the anonymity and invisibilization surrounding the working classes, in particular care workers, and an individuality lost to colonial dispossession.

The enduring instability and indeterminacy of the names of many Black people in French society at the time originates from the practices of naming the enslaved. The act of invalidation of the names of enslaved populations born in Africa is the first sign of dispossession of their individuality because one's first name retains, scholar Priska Degras contends in her 2011 study about the significance of proper names in literatures from the Americas, "[la] modalité de distinction, de reconnaissance et d'appartenance" (the mode of distinction, of recognition and of belonging) (10). The subsequent act of renaming by the slave owner is in that context meant to assert dominance in all forms over the existence of enslaved people. For Glissant, "the African deported by the Middle Passage" is "the naked migrant [*le migrant nu*]" as they arrive in the Caribbean and the Americas with "only the traces of [their] original country" (2008, 87).[17] For indeed, made-up first names and nicknames assigned to the enslaved pertain to a system of oppression designed to maintain class, racial, and social domination. Again, when slavery was abolished for the second time on April 27, 1848, first and family names were given to newly affranchised populations, reenacting the exclusive white privilege of naming. In his novel *Le quatrième siècle*, Édouard Glissant explores in particular the immense symbolism of power resting on the act of naming, as cited by Degras in *L'obsession du nom dans le roman des Amériques* (2011):

> Ils acceptaient que tu portes un nom, à condition qu'ils te le donnent. S'ils avaient décidé pour La Pointe, va donc leur faire admettre que tu veux Longué, à cause que Longué est comme un dongré de farine bien pris dans un bouillon de crabes et raide comme un bois campeche. Va donc leur faire admettre! Que ton nom est pour toi, choisi par toi? Ils n'acceptent pas! . . . si dans d'autres cas—quand tu osais en choisir un et décidais de le porter toi seul—ils t'auraient tué pour te l'ôter sans retour. Ils

décrétaient alors: "Il n'a aucun droit à porter ce nom." Sauf encore, si le nom les flattait. (1964, 166)

They were perfectly willing for you to have a name provided they gave it to you. If they had decided on La-Pointe, just try and make them acknowledge that you want Longoué, because Longoué is like a good, solid ash-cake in crab soup, and unbending as a campeche tree. Get them to stand for it! That your name is for you and chosen by you? They'll never agree! . . . even if in other cases—when you dared choose one and decided on your own that it was yours—they would have killed you just to take it irrevocably away. Then they would proclaim: "He has no right at all to have a name." Except, again, if the name was flattering to them. (2001, 167–168)

The act of unnaming performed by the slaveholder paired with the loss of the privilege of naming for the enslaved makes the social and racial power dynamics legible in colonial times. In a contemporary context then, what is in the act of renaming, of claiming to individualize once nameless others? In other words, who receives care in the act of renaming conducted by the Paris *Modèle noir* exhibition's curators?

As I have discussed, the *Modèle noir* exhibition's main intent is described as an effort to shift from type to individual—that is, to assume the role of repairing, of giving care to injured subjectivities. But because the renaming is conditional on limited historical documentation, the interpretation is bound to be questionable unless it can engage with the processes of erasure that linked the circumstances and life experiences of Black people to slavery, colonialism, and care economies. These processes clearly affected what was recorded and how it was recorded at the time. Curators' battles against erasure echo, in a way, French literary scholar Alexandre Gefen's critical outlook on twentieth-century literature which would "faire de l'Histoire ni une toile de fond ni une force obscure mais un discours à redresser par des renarrations complémentaires et correctrices" (make History neither a background nor a dark force, but a discourse able to correct through additional and corrective retellings) (2018, 235). Although the attempt at retrospective repairing cannot be denied, I am questioning the pathway toward an assumed and possibly imposed rehabilitation of the silenced voices of colonial France.

Put differently, due to an unshakable process of erasure, attempts to repair are in most cases limited to the unstable renaming of once nameless others—renaming that is nonetheless carried out by the exhibition's curators. The polysemy of the term "model" is, for them, fit for the purpose of historical rehabilitation as it can refer to both "[l']individu regardé, représenté par l'artiste" (the individual seen, represented by the artist) but also "modèle porteur de valuers" (model bearer of values). And yet the lives of Black models, irrevocably entangled with the structures of knowledge production that have produced their anonymity, are generally accompanied with a question mark—their lives summed up in a first name or a nickname. It seems here that caring does not so much concern the presumed receivers of care (the Black models), but rather the alleged caregivers (the exhibition's curators, enthusiastic museum-goers, French society at large?) who can maybe rejoice in the cathartic act of "redressing" the damage while avoiding, consciously or not, the fractures inherited from colonialism and slavery.

Our ability to reconstitute the lives trapped in a system of erasure is compromised by the structures of knowledge production that generated their absence, as I have just demonstrated through my study of the *Modèle noir* exhibitions. The way in which they peripherally appear in what Marisa Fuentes calls "the traditional archive," which has been formed by "the majority of documents produced during the era of slavery . . . by colonial administrators, planters, white men and women, and governing in the metropole" (Owens 2016, 7), reveals their invisibilized, silenced, and objectified existence. The prevalent economic discourse surrounding the lives of the colonized means that much has been left out or erased from the "traditional" archival documents. It also means that we inherit "archival obscurity" (Morgan 2021, 9) and illegibility.

The opacity shrouding the enslaved's history is precisely the challenge writer Fabienne Kanor confronts, opening the novel *Humus* (2006; English translation 2020) with her personal realization of the scarce, incomplete, and objectifying historical accounts surrounding the lives of the enslaved. During a visit to the Archives Départementales of the city of Nantes in France, Kanor read about an incident that took place in 1774 aboard the slave ship *Le Soleil*: fourteen unnamed African women escaped the ship's hold and leaped overboard, all together, to resist their enslavement. Only six of them survived while the others drowned or were killed by sharks. Kanor reproduces the report of the incident in the logbook of the ship's captain, Louis Mosnier, which reads as follows:

> On the 23rd of March last, fourteen Black women apparently leaped overboard, from the poop deck into the sea, all together in one movement. Despite all possible diligence, with the sea extremely choppy and the wind blowing a gale, sharks had already eaten several of them before any could be hauled back on board, yet seven were saved, one of whom died that evening at seven o'clock, being in very bad shape when rescued, so in the end, eight were lost in the incident. (2020, 7)

The captain's technical discourse abounds in lifeless numbers, stressing economic loss while silencing these women's collective (in the sense of all at the same time) act of "suicidal resistance" (Calhoun 2021, 132). "How to tell, how to retell this story told by men?" Kanor asks (2020, 9). How, indeed?

Kanor simultaneously grapples with the limitations, the historical lacunae of traditional archives produced within an ideological system where constructed racial hierarchy places the captive Africans in the category of human merchandise and labor force, while also challenging such ordering of human lives. Motivated by "a desire to swap," "to trade away technical discourse for the spoken word," Kanor's writing makes us reflect on ways to revitalize the flattened, disembodied experiences of individual women by, at the same time, spurring awareness of the historical plundering of individual identities and making visible the lasting impact of that oppression (2020, 9). Kanor exposes at once the materiality of the archive (Louis Mosnier's report) while also exposing its fallibility, making space for frustration, shock, pain, and disbelief to be expressed and prompting the disavowal of the authority of the traditional archive. I wish, then, to demonstrate the possibility of transmuting through the fictional the "archival obscurity" into productive opacity, the unified and consigned into the incomplete and ruptured. Ultimately, I am interested in highlighting the tension between the acts of repairing and of caregiving, and our responsibility in the act of reckoning with the historically obscured, silenced, and abused lives of the colonized.

Through the etymological investigation of the word "archive," French philosopher Jacques Derrida highlights that the term comes from the Greek *Arkhé* which means both "origin" (*le commencement*) and "rule" (*le commandement*). The archive, then, is historically constructed as a center of power, serving a crucial function of recording and organizing what has been admitted as archival materials by archivists (*archontes*). Anything, at first, is archivable; but cultural objects and texts become *archives* following the archival processing they undergo in a totalizing gesture. Archivists, in this configuration, are record managers and keepers, "gather[ing] the functions of unification, of identification, of classification" paired with "the power of consignation" (Derrida 1995, 10). Consignation is here defined by Derrida in terms of *"gathering together signs"* in the written form, aiming to "coordinate a single corpus, in a system or a synchrony in which all the elements articulate the unity of an ideal configuration." The ordering principle specific to the traditional archive is, for instance, what we see expressed in the captain's original report. Instead, Kanor's narrative strategy in

Humus challenges the material realities and limitations of this document by fabricating twelve narratives told in the first person by successive female speakers designated by a definite noun that captures only a piece of who they were: "La muette," "La vieille," "L'esclave," L'amazone," "La blanche," "Les jumelles" (two distinct voices in the text), "L'employée," "La petite," "La reine," "La volante," "La mère," and "L'héritière." The organization of the novel in titled sections thus swaps the indefinite, numerical plural of the captain's anecdotal report for the singular plural, meaning that the group of women act collectively to resist their enslavement, but the text makes their individual experiences and subjectivities perfectly visible. In *Humus*, the production of individual (though relational) experiences resorts to the opacity and unavailability of memory around these fourteen anonymous captives, equipping "le décalage . . . entre le document d'archive et l'imagination de l'écrivain" (the gap . . . between the archival document and the writer's imagination) (Lionnet 2021, quoted in in Jean-François 2017) with the capacity to construct "an alternative archival fragment" (Francis 2016, 70). Here, the fictional is driven by the responsibility to care, inciting forms of attention to silenced voices.

The transmutation of opacity into fictional fabric in *Humus* provides an opportunity to interrogate the intersection of care and literature. This inquiry, as previously outlined in the introduction, remains fairly open-ended, ripe for further examination. Hence, what does giving care in or through literature imply here? How do we navigate the textual pathways of caregiving textually while also acknowledging the potential obstacles that may hinder it? More precisely, I am interested in questioning the meanings and gestures of care that emerge at the intersection of caregiving and historical acts of colonial erasure in light of Kanor's treatment of the voices of the fourteen captives.

In her analysis of *Humus* in her book-length study *Odious Caribbean Women and the Palpable Aesthetics of Transgression* (2017), scholar Gladys M. Francis places the emphasis on the writing of the body, the "process of writing that literally—gives *body* to;

embodies; gives presence to—a *body*" (xvii, emphases in original). Although it is true that Kanor's response to her encounter with objectified bodies in the archives is to "give presence" to the captives, the condition of their "embodied corporeality" (Kanor 2020, 69) is, I will argue, to claim a voice, to speak again. At the beginning of the narrative, Kanor insists on the act of listening, the commitment to hearing that befalls us: "Like these shadowy figures put in chains long ago, the reader is condemned not to move from this moment on. Just *listen* with no other distraction to this chorus of women. At the risk of losing your bearings, *hear* once more these hearts beating" (2020, 9, emphasis mine). Their coming into existence, then, occurs in language, through voice. In her philosophical exploration of subjecthood, French philosopher Sandra Laugier argues that voice is what defines the subject: having, using voice is about "*being alive*" (2015, 74, emphasis in original). In effect, the suppression of voice negates the foundation of the individual as a subject. Thus, with no voice to claim, the subject is made absent—becoming a voiceless body. What we see challenged in *Humus* is the historical making of voicelessness, and also expressed is the reclaiming of a voice to listen to and to reckon with.

Describing the writing of *Humus*, Kanor points to the reinsertion of voice: "les voix d'autrefois [qui] n'ont pas fini de nous parler" (voices from the past [that] have not finished talking to us) (Herbeck 2013, 967). For indeed, Kanor adds, "il n'y a pas un mot de ce roman qui n'ait été chanté, murmuré ou répété à haute voix plusieurs fois" (there is not a single word of this novel that has not been sung, whispered or repeated aloud multiple times) (Herbeck 2013, 968). In the face of "la mort de la parole" (the death of the spoken word) (Kanor 2006, 14; 2020, 9), the fictional takes over for these fourteen women to regain voice and to speak again, for the writer to bring them into the conversation, and for us to listen to voices that have been denied existence. As such, the fictional creates space for speaking and listening to take place, pluralmindedly but not necessarily cohesively or in a linear manner. These very different women's voices, as Doyle Calhoun observes, "have forgotten names, places, dates"; "they fail to remember, choose not to remember, or remember imperfectly. They try to forget. They fabricate, invent, and lie" (2021, 134).

The figure of "La muette" (the Mute Woman), who opens the narrative, is a potent indicator of the difficulty of excavating the voice, the challenge of finding what to say in the face of absence, of telling the made-absent and the invisibilized. The Mute Woman, then, opens the novel with the recognition that she, along with the other women captives, was denied a voice and is grappling with what it is she wants to say. "I saw everything. Don't ask me what. Lost words are lost forever" (Kanor 2020, 13)—the possibility to alert to the historical circumstances of erasure ("I saw everything") is here immediately contained by the silencing of voices under the violence of colonial rule ("Lost words are lost forever"). These women's voices are therefore presented struggling, hesitant, at times rambling and cryptic. Throughout, the language of the text is, in effect, interrogative ("Ohé! Has anyone seen my name?" says the Mute Woman; Kanor 2020, 17); stammered ("Moldy, me vomited, spoiled, thrown away. Me rancid. Dirty. Salty. Without. Alone," says "La Blanche"; Kanor 2020, 90); discontinued both temporally (before their capture, aboard the ship, and the times after that) and spatially (where they come from, where they are, and for some where they will be).

In the process, these voices, long held in silence, recover, via the fictional, the ability to speak for themselves while also challenging the limitations on the enslaved body. In fact, these women captives occasionally evidence the necessary parting from the materiality of their bodies. In this instance, the material body is what ties their existence to gendered and hypersexualized assumptions as well as to the numerical rationality of the slave system—the technical archival practices that the captain of *Le Soleil*'s report exemplifies. La Blanche, who loses her mind after having survived the leap into the sea ("After that, I went mad"; 2020, 85), tells of her own suicide on the plantation; as she recounts her body being found, her voice becomes spectral as though emanating from beyond corporeality: "They found me at dawn. In the back of the workshop, in the big room where they wring juice from the cane. They say it wasn't a pretty sight, all that blood on the workbench ... I was galloping, I—blanche, the body ravaged. A dress without ruffle or thread. Vast. Finally free" (2020, 121). Such an imaginary flight from corporeal enslavement both resists the ideological rationalization that produces commodified Black bodies as part of the slave system and releases the voice.

Now let us recall the contested pathway toward historical rehabilitation of silenced and objectified bodies in the context of the *Modèle noir* exhibition, which suggests this rehabilitation can be achieved through the combination of an attempt at giving a name and the display of "individual" bodies. Even if the project might be driven by a notion of care, the emphasis placed on *re-*embodiment establishes the shift from the unknown to the known as the sole mode of interaction with unreckoned colonial practices of erasure. The way the exhibition is organized around categories such as "les nourrices noires" (Black nannies) shows how bodies of knowledge are produced at a given time, but also, perhaps inadvertently, how we perpetuate them into the present. By way of example, the museum note for the section "Les nourrices noires" reads as follows: "Au XIXe siècle, les femmes noires sont particulièrement recherchées comme nourrices par les familles de la haute société, leur lait étant réputé d'excellente qualité. Ces usages, parfois raillés par la caricature, étaient déjà ceux de l'aristocratie dans les colonies sous l'Ancien Régime" (In the nineteenth century, Black women were keenly sought after as wet nurses by high-society families because their milk had a reputation for being of an excellent quality. This practice, which was sometimes mocked in caricatures, was prevalent among the aristocracy in the colonies during the Ancien Régime). The language surrounding the depicted women not only reveals a moment in the organization of knowledge, information, and power (the ability to assign a particular social category) in the past but also as it is reproduced at the time of the exhibition. The way the lives of "the Black nannies" are accounted for here follows the same ordering as when pictures of European modern life are being produced. That is, we find expressed in the museum discourse the same essentializing and stereotypical qualities used to lay out the terms of their past existence, also establishing their object status, their silent embodiment.

Contrary to adopting generalizing identity markers, Kanor elucidates her writing process,

> Mon intention n'était ni de magnifier ni de "gonfler" mes personnages pour en faire des emblèmes, des porte-histoires. Je n'ai pas écrit ce roman pour dénoncer "les affres de l'esclavage"; c'eût été candide et parfaitement inutile. J'ai tout simplement voulu conter l'histoire d'Africaines mises en fer, mais qui continuent d'être des femmes, elles vieillissent, elles attendent leurs règles, elles se chamaillent, elles se racontent des histoires, elles se souviennent, elles pensent à leur homme, elles tombent malades, folles ou bien amoureuses. (Herbeck 2013, 970)

> My intent was neither to idealize nor to "amplify" my characters to turn them into symbols, bearers of history. I have not written this novel to denounce slavery; that would have been naive and completely useless. I simply wanted to tell the story of African women put in chains, but who continue to be women, they grow old, they have their period, they bicker, they tell each other stories, they reminisce, they think of their man, they fall sick, into madness, or in love.

In effect, Kanor's writing disrupts the continuum of colonial time by challenging the *order of things*; and by flirting with the possibility of disruption, she presents the possibility for things to get messy. Throughout *Humus*, the women's voices talk over each other, dialog with each other, and quibble, perhaps then echoing the amplification of voices that Kanor hints at in her interview with Jason Herbeck.

For instance, La Blanche reacts disapprovingly to the name she was given by the other captives: "La Blanche. That's what they call me. What they say when they think I can't hear them. La Blanche and a lot of other names, too. Words that soil, ruin my name" (Kanor 2020, 73). She might have got this nickname because she had lighter skin, as we learn from the twins (2020, 98), or it may be because she consented to sexual relations with a sailor to win him over (though he eventually turns away from her after she tells him she is pregnant). Though she maintains "[she] couldn't care less what they think," La Blanche clearly hears her fellow captives' critical voices and cares enough to engage with them, even if it means to disagree (2020, 73). In any case, instances of La Blanche's self-expression challenge the ways in which she is perceived by the others, insisting that she is guided by her own sense of self-preservation. "For me, I believe there are days when you just don't have the choice.... And I, La Blanche, have decided not to die" (2020, 73). Although her attitude may be perceived as treacherous or submissive, the character reinserts her own voice ("I, La Blanche") and speaks for herself.

The Little One adds a contrasting perspective on La Blanche because she lacks an understanding about the meaning of her nickname; instead, she calls her "the Grown-up," reflecting the bond that has grown between the two. La Blanche performs the different roles within the Little One's vision of a family structure: "She's happy to be my sister, the Grown-up. Or father, or mother. Whatever I wish" (2020, 116). The Slave similarly equates self-expression with solipsism as the subject is claimed through the use of voice. The character's section of the narrative is punctuated with the words "I, daughter of Nupe, I" followed by an active verb: "I, small daughter of Nupe, I love" (2020, 50), she says when she tells of her love for another woman also held captive in the barracoons. To express her love for this woman is to act against the dominant order, "the Law" (2020, 50). This means of self-assertion is a sign of her nascent expressivity.

I now want to turn back to Laugier's definition of the subject as voice. In redefining the subject through the subjectivity of language defined by voice, Laugier explains that to have a voice means to lose it to an Other because "expression itself as life form" is "a life that is not mine anymore" (2015, 78). In other words, in a situation where I speak to someone, I consent to being heard—my voice being realized when someone engages with what is expressed. As such, Kanor creates a fictional space where voices of the enslaved can exist. Within that space, expressions of agreement or disagreement between the different characters are the sign that self-expressivity and attention to that expressiveness are made possible. Given the emphasis on the first person, the path toward self-expressivity for the women characters who populate the text is thus focused on the individuals and their particular circumstances. For instance, Kanor writes the character of "the Employee," "une captive à demi" (a half captive) (Herbeck 2013, 969), whose father was a boatman and who works as a guard on *Le Soleil*. Tasked with watching the prisoners, when she sees "the thirteen rebels" getting ready to jump, "something broke inside [her]. [She] wanted to be like them. They were so beautiful. With no hesitation, she jumped" (Kanor 2020, 111). The way the female characters of *Humus* are voiced steers clear of a narrative of undifferentiated collective resistance where they would act toward a common goal (i.e., freedom from slavery). Instead, the characters are not always squarely oppositional: for example, the Amazon rallies the women and will later join a Maroon community; the Employee joins them spontaneously before going back to work on a Portuguese ship; the Queen allies herself with the rebels after the Amazon has promised her that she will help her conquer her kingdom again; and the list goes on.

In an interview with Emily A. Owens to discuss her book *Dispossessed Lives: Enslaved Women, Violence and the Archive* (2016), Fuentes signals the problem of agency in relation to binary models where the enslaved are portrayed as either victims or fighters. "The historiography of slavery," Fuentes contends, "ha[s] been influenced by the political project of telling heroic (and often masculinist) narratives of resistance and triumph" (Owens 2016, answer 4). Fuentes's scholarly project offers different methodological examples such as "incomplete narratives, non-conforming structures, and different modes of writing" to challenge historical linearity and make visible instead "the complicated forms of representation" of enslaved women's experiences and Caribbean slavery in general (Owens 2016, answer 1). This being said, Fuentes makes her intervention clear: she is not creating fiction. In the case of Kanor, by contrast, incompleteness is what spurs fictional creation.

By giving shape to the character of "the Heiress," Kanor endows the act of fictional creation with the responsibility to excavate voices from the damaged form in which these enslaved women appear in archival records. As Kanor writes herself into the heiress, her writing practice interrogates absence and questions what language to use to represent these women's complicated forms of existence, the means of expression with which to equip these voices retrieved from forced silence. For example, when the heiress describes her trip to Badagry and the Door of No Return in Nigeria, in frustration she demands answers from a landscape of historical silencing. Studying fading footprints in the sand, she asks, "Where did they lead? Back to the days of hunters and Black-captive-eating-sharks, two centuries ago? . . . Had I done the right thing, coming here? Would this beach tell me any more than the blank page?" (2020, 174). The questions hang in the air, entrusting the heiress with the responsibility to imagine, through fiction, the different voices that may emanate from the violence of historical erasure. Such writing practice means to be attentive to the limits of historical representation while capturing the voices long silenced, bringing them into focus.

In fact, by naming herself the Heiress, the writer, the first-person narrator, first accepts as true the inheritance passed on to her; only after that does she accept what has been inherited (i.e., the violence of the archive and of the erasure of the experiences of the enslaved). The generic definition of the substantive "heir" or "heiress" includes a focus on the act of receiving something—tangible or intangible *assets*: an heir or heiress is "one who receives property from an ancestor, one who is entitled to inherit property," or "one who inherits or is entitled to succeed to a hereditary rank, title, or office."[18] From this definition we understand that, through the process of inheritance, there may be something to be "gained" in the economic or social sense of added "value."

As for debt, in a Western context and in the financial sense, what is owed generally does not fall under the responsibility of surviving relatives—as such, one is, unless in special circumstances, not held accountable for what is absent, what remains incomplete. Thus, such understanding of the distribution of inheritance admits first that the heir or heiress has no responsibility toward the debt, and then that what has not been settled is just lost. The heiress in *Humus* contrasts with the standard configuration of inheritance in that she accepts responsibility toward the absent. The absence of tangible evidence surrounding the lives of the enslaved, which translates into a debt, becomes the heiress's legacy—an absence she employs to "represent the lives of the nameless and the forgotten, ... reckon[ing] with loss, and ... respect[ing] the limits of what cannot be known" (Hartman 2008, 4). By grappling with the heritability of historical erasure, the Heiress confronts not only the past lives of the enslaved steeped in silence but also the persistence of that silence (and silencing) in the present. "Je regrette d'être venue, r'grette d'être venue, gret'd'v'nue" ("I'm sorry I came, sorry I came, sorryIcame") (Kanor 2006, 240; 2020, 181)—the language of the *papa-feuilles*, the healer, is disorderly, fragmented, and in difficulty, just like the voices that come into existence throughout the text, alerting to the devastating effect of erasure but also battling to imagine what forms of care to give in order to move forward.

In the English translation of the novel by Lynn E. Palermo, the term "papa-feuilles" is, in fact, annotated: when the narrator visits the studio of her artist friend, Pietr-Pedro-Pierre-Peter (his name changes each time), she finds herself surrounded by "her papers." Or perhaps "were they the leaves of the tree [of forgetfulness]" that the men captives had to go around nine times and the women captives seven times because this would supposedly make them forget where they came from (2020, 186)?[19] The novel-to-be, the paralyzing blank pages are in the beginning soaked in silence, that of the archives but also that of the sea. Then, after that, there are words—that is, voice—"the cry, too long contained, muffled by the song of the seas and all the discourse of men" (2020, 187). In the studio space, Peter then whispers to the Heiress in the concluding moments of the novel, "Nous sommes des papas-feuilles" ("We are the *papa-feuilles*, the healers") (2006, 247; 2020, 187), as the narrator-writer attempts to attend to the dispersed leaves of the Tree.

Although there is no direct equivalent to capture the cultural specificity of the "*papa-feuilles*," Palermo's annotation conveys the particularities of reparative practices rooted in the knowledge of medicinal plants passed on from generation to generation in Afro-Caribbean contexts. "In the Caribbean as well as in Africa," scholar Renée Larrier explains, "certain roots—as in plants, bark and leaves—are prescribed for therapeutic purposes.... In Caribbean literature [in turn] 'racines-médecine' and its practitioners are an essential weapon against illness and disease" (1998, 87). Clearly here we steer clear of any derogatory interpretation of healing practices, which were feared, Larrier reminds us, by French owners who "were terrified of being poisoned" by Africans deported to the Americas (1998, 87). Rather, through her writing, the Heiress transforms productively the way in which the papa-feuilles's ability to heal, to repair, manifests itself as the narrator manipulates humus, the opaque material resulting from the degradation of the lives of the enslaved; she formulates a caring gesture that accounts for the nonelucidated and damaged, the incomplete and fragmented which must inform the narratives around the colonial past and its legacy we tell in the present.

The commitment to memorialize the forgotten and the missing, evident in Kanor's *Humus*, serves to commemorate what persists as unknown and will continue to remain so. The portrayal of historical opacity does not diminish the significance of individual enslaved lives; instead, it bears witness to the difficulty of recovery and caregiving. What the curatorial discourses around the *Modèle noir* exhibitions seek to achieve is restitution through text of what was initially denied, beginning with something as fundamental as a name or a tangible trace in archival records. However, it may not be possible to redress anonymity—especially not through conjecture and the replacement of racial terms—in order to alleviate the violence of the erasure of enslaved and colonized lives. It appears that practices of care stemming from such an insurmountable past may originate from the acceptance of an inherited absence. Efforts to attend to and represent the absence may therefore require the seeking of ways of inhabiting the gap, suspended in midair alongside Kanor's fourteen captives—not entirely vanished, yet not entirely present either.

2

Voices of the BUMIDOM, or the Colonial Legacy of Care Work

In *Lettres à une Noire*, Françoise Ega, a Martinican woman who moved to Marseille in the 1950s with her children and husband, reflects on the migration of Antilleans to hexagonal France from the early 1960s onward: "Est-ce la traite? Est-ce la traite qui recommence?" (Is it the slave trade? Is it the slave trade that is starting again?) (1978, 58). Ega writes more particularly about the plight of Antillean women who were typically employed to work as maids (especially live-in) in white bourgeois households during that time period. In point of fact, such domestic industry became integral to a much wider system of placements in the sectors of manual labor and construction (mostly for men) and domestic service and public hospitals (mostly for women) as part of the Bureau pour le Développement des Migrations dans les Départements d'Outre-Mer (BUMIDOM, the Office for the Development of the Migration in the Overseas Departments), a state-regulated agency created by Michel Debré (deputy for Réunion between 1963 and 1988).[1] Between the years 1963 and 1982, close to 200,000 individuals from Réunion (76, 583), Guadeloupe (63,505), Martinique (43,516), and French Guiana (2,685) emigrated to hexagonal France after being granted a one-way ticket through the BUMIDOM.[2]

Written between the years 1962 and 1964 when the BUMIDOM was being implemented, Ega's epistolary diary, *Lettres à une Noire*, though published posthumously in 1978, probes the making of a racialized and gendered assignment to caring labor for Antillean women coming to work in hexagonal France at the time. In her *Lettres*, she imagines a one-sided epistolary conversation with Carolina Maria de Jesus, a Black Brazilian woman who lived in the favela of Canindé, São Paulo, with her children, and who is also the author of the memoir *Child of the Dark* (1960). Ega relates to Carolina, whose struggle through poverty has affected her (Ega read a digest about Carolina's life in the magazine *Paris Match*) and with whom she stands, or rather writes, in imagined solidarity.[3]

In *Child of the Dark*, Carolina Maria de Jesus recounts in the first-person her daily challenges as a single mother with limited resources, striving to raise her three children in a favela between the years 1955 and 1958. In her memoir, she also mentions her passion for literature and her decision to eventually write the story of her own life. Although Ega had not read Carolina's book, she found in the portrayal of her life a kindred spirit, resonating with the struggles of Antillean women in France. Indeed, Ega confides to Carolina her investigation into the life of a care worker from the perspective of an Antillean woman. After seeking a job as a household worker in the service of white bourgeois families from Marseille, Ega began to write about the abuse of those she calls her "sisters," disrupting a hierarchy of attention linked to that of domestic service as well as speaking against the silences surrounding the BUMIDOM.

There has so far been substantial investigation into the BUMIDOM's purported goals—scholars such as Alain Anselin (1979), Audrey Célestine (2018), Stéphanie Condon and Celia Britton (2020), Anny Dominique Curtius (2010), Félix Germain (2010), H. Adlai Murdoch (2020), Pap Ndiaye (2008), Sylvain Pattieu (2016, 2021), and Antonia Wimbush (2018, 2022), among others, have taken up the task of elucidating the historical, political, and socioeconomic contexts surrounding the creation of the state agency. All agree that through the BUMIDOM the French government consciously attempted conjointly to furnish a profitable and exploitable labor pool in the postwar period, to curb rural depopulation, and to eliminate social movements, especially among unionized, anticolonialist, and separatist youth, which were gaining momentum by the end of the 1950s in the overseas departments.[4] An expanding corpus—documentary and fictional—that I allude to in part throughout this chapter provides insight into the wide range of affective experiences of those who left through the BUMIDOM and their descendants.[5]

But the BUMIDOM experience itself remains largely shrouded in silence. That silence exists in layers. There initially was silence about the decision to come to hexagonal France to find work with the BUMIDOM. For example, in the documentary film *L'avenir est ailleurs* (The future is elsewhere; Maestrati 2007) the process of departure with the BUMIDOM is reconstituted in the fictional character of Timothée Bolo, who is preparing to leave home to work as a housekeeper in hexagonal France. In the sequence preceding her boarding the boat, her uncle tells her to not answer when her name is called but rather to embark "comme tout le monde" (like everybody else) as if she were "une grande voyageuse" (well-traveled). The example of Antoine-Léonard Maestrati's film reveals in particular that a presumed or known association with the program may have caused shame at the time, for it suggested that economic survival had become dependent on a constricted overseas-hexagonal France mobility.

The migratory experience was originally marked by some form of secrecy that over time became an inherited silence around the conditions of departure as well as arrival in the Hexagon. For indeed, we see also that after they have arrived in France some migrants would keep the reality of their situation quiet. Charlise Curier writes in *Mon aventure avec le BUMIDOM* that she emigrated to France in 1971 and was sent to the "la Tour" center in Crouy-sur-Ourcq, in the Seine-et-Marne department to be trained to become a "femm[e] de ménage" (housekeeper), "*voire* [une] servant[e]" (or even a maid) (31). There, she explains, "je ne racontais pas à mes parents tout ce que je vivais. Je ne voulais pas leur faire de la peine" (I would not tell my parents what I was going through. I did not want to hurt them) (33). It is then easy for that past to slip into self-repressed memories, unattended histories, and distant knowledge. They create a seeming absence that Curier attempts to fix partially, decades later, by telling her own story with the BUMIDOM.

Following this quiet generation of BUMIDOM travelers, it is not rare to find discontinued familial memory either due to the relative silence surrounding this migration or the detachment of the next generation, usually individuals born in the Hexagon.[6] Building on the existence of an already persistent silence among BUMIDOM migrants, I start this chapter by exploring the complicity of caring labor (i.e., domestic service) in constituting en masse a BUMIDOM-specific invisibilized workforce in the context of Ega's epistolary diary, *Lettres à une Noire* ([1978] 2021; hereafter *LN*). An analysis of Ega's writing in the first part of this chapter helps analyze the making of a naturalized hierarchy of service in the context of the BUMIDOM, which eventually consolidates asymmetrical forms of attention on the basis of class, gender, and race. Writing her personal account of the domestic service, Ega writes in reaction to such hierarchical models.

In light of the time period, Ega's writing becomes undoubtedly set against the backdrop of the BUMIDOM years, although the state-run program is only mentioned a couple of times throughout the narrative and once is even reported, perhaps intentionally, under the incorrect name "Zubidom" by a friend of Ega living in Paris (*LN*, 185). The implicit presence of the BUMIDOM exacerbates the making of silence and invisibility that eventually defines the French Caribbean migration through the agency. For Ega, to write was, I argue, not only to refuse implicitly the silence around the BUMIDOM but more importantly to develop kinds of attention that focus on the experiences of caregivers, her "sisters," rather than on those who disproportionately demand care (the *patrons* and *patronnes*). In keeping with an emphasis on shifting forms of attention, the second half of this chapter provides an analysis of *Péyi an nou* (Kreyòl for "our country"; 2017; hereafter *PN*), a graphic narrative by Jessica Oublié (scenarist) and Marie-Ange Rousseau (illustrator) that gives us a more general insight into the quiet memories of the BUMIDOM, making them emerge in the present day.[7] Through the interplay between the structure of the BUMIDOM and the distribution of caregiving, this chapter places care work within the legacies of colonialism and slavery while also analyzing the formal expressions in literary and graphic texts that emphasize voices of the BUMIDOM.

Framing the effacement of the BUMIDOM through the lens of caring labor brings into focus an inherently formed invisibility; this invisibility is tied not only to the kinds of tasks performed but also to the historical and social distribution of domestic service. As broadly defined by Camille Barbagallo and Silvia Federici (2012), domestic work is a particular aspect of reproductive labor, which includes the performance of tasks such as housecleaning, laundry, cooking, and other supportive tasks by family members or hired workers—a form of labor that implies caring in the sense that it aims to shape and maintain a living and livable environment. In developing a conceptual understanding of care work, theorists such as Caroline Ibos, Sandra Laugier, Pascale Molinier, and Patricia Paperman, among others,[8] have described care work as what goes on without being seen—a set of tasks whose completion relies on them not being noticed when satisfyingly performed. More specific to housekeeping, Molinier points that "housework, [if] it is well done, should not be seen and should not disturb the daily life of whoever is benefitting from it, otherwise it has failed" (292).[9] On the basis of such conditions for success, caring labor puts the caregiver at risk.

For one might be tempted to wish for a "subjectless care" (Molinier, 296), and the concurrent dehumanization of the caregiver is always more or less a probability. In fact, in *Lettres (LN)*, Ega observes her own depersonalization process when she starts working as a housekeeper in wealthy homes of Marseille. She describes, for example, that despite having worked for the same family for fifteen days, no one had yet asked for her name or her identity card; she is reduced only to the role of the maid. She notes indeed that her *patrons* show no interest in who she is outside the function she occupies in their home: "Je suis la bonne" (I am the maid), Ega sums up. After a year of employment, Ega comments her transformation into an "engin corvéable" (an exploited machine) (*LN*, 175), to the point of assimilating the body, which has become object, to the instrument of labor. Her body now reflects the difficult and arduous nature of the work she accomplishes. "Il y a une chose qui ne peut se camoufler, les mains, elles sont les cartes de visite des individus" (There is one thing that cannot be hidden. Hands give away someone's occupation), as Ega depicts the state of her hands. She goes on, "Aujourd'hui les miennes sont sans ongles, ou presque, et toutes plissées malgré la couche de glycérine que j'y ai passée" (Today I don't have any nails left, or barely, and my hands are wrinkly in spite of the layer of glycerin I apply) (*LN*, 189). Paradoxically, work that is expected to be "invisible" leaves an indelible visibility on the suffering body of those who carry out the labor of caring, irrevocably linking their physical identity with the tasks performed.

Even more pronounced is the pernicious idea of "invisible work" when it becomes integrated into the shaping of the BUMIDOM labor pool, wherein migrant workers are groomed for low-paid and socially marginalizing work. The emblematic BUMIDOM training center located in Crouy-sur-Ourcq, which Curier mentions in *Mon aventure avec le BUMIDOM*, was instrumental in solidifying a racialized, gendered, and geographically determined distribution of care work.[10] *Péyi an Nou* (Oublié and Rousseau 2017) emphasizes this aspect. One panel in particular recounts the typical journey of an individual arriving with the BUMIDOM, as it was explained to Oublié and Rousseau by late anthropologist Alain

Anselin (Figure 1): placements with the BUMIDOM led to either immediate employment for people with qualifications or, for people with no identified qualifications, transfer to the training centers. These were known as the FPA, or Centre de Formation Professionnelle pour Adultes (Professional Training Center for Adults, also called the Centre d'Adaptation à la Vie Métropolitaine, the Adaptation Center to Metropolitan Life) (*PN*, 127). We see in the case of nonqualified BUMIDOM candidates two possible alternatives marked by an arrow: in the bottom panel, on a map of France, the first arrow indicates Simandres, located in the Rhône department; the second arrow points to Crouy-sur-Ourcq. To the left of the map, a Black male figure sits on a workout bench lifting weights—the Simandres center prepared Antillean men for employment in construction, metallurgy, and machine industries. To the right of the map, we see a Black female subject dressed as maid; a mop and bucket appear in a splash icon adjacent to her, almost unexpectedly—emanata lines are shown close to her head to signal surprise or shock.

In fact, the relegation of Antillean women to domestic service was not limited to supposedly "unskilled" individuals: in *L'avenir est ailleurs*, during an interview with the Clérence family in Le Gosier, Guadeloupe, Faustina Clérence reveals that despite her qualifications as a schoolteacher, she was offered a job as a maid after she arrived in the Hexagon. Employment through the BUMIDOM clearly did not meet the hopes of upward social mobility of those leaving; rather, the program played a central role in the shaping of a workforce from the overseas departments who were specifically mass-trained to join the service and care industry—a framework "they had been trying to escape" by coming to the Hexagon, Murdoch rightly notes.[11]

Péyi an nou is again useful in showing the disillusionment linked to a deceitful recruitment process. Two panels are here juxtaposed: on the left panel, we see a young woman, at home, hand clasped in the hope of training to become a doctor after she arrives in France;

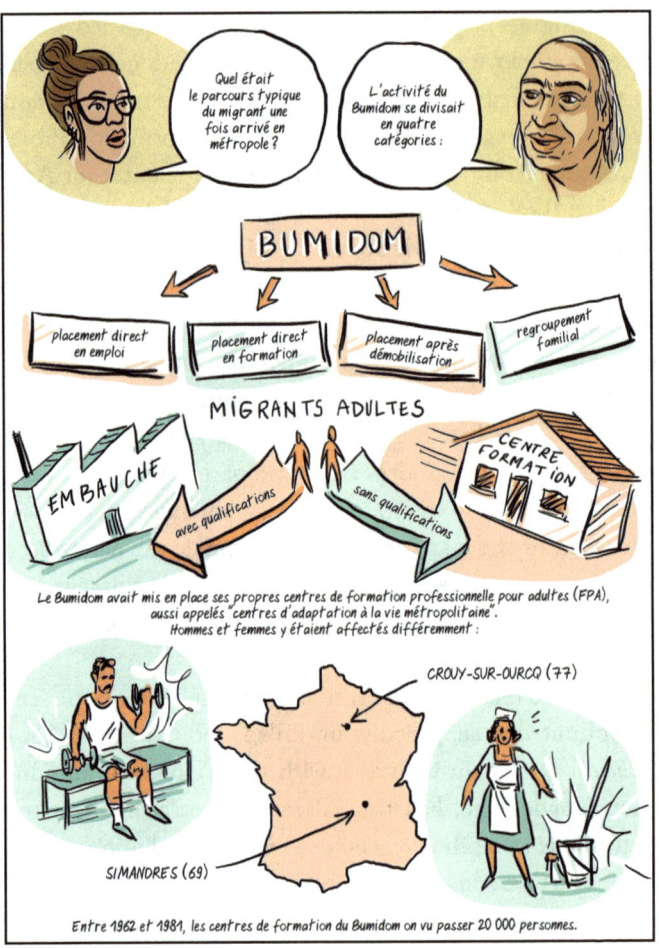

FIG. 1. *Péyi an nou*, page 127 © Steinkis, 2024.

Text from left to right, and in the order of appearance:

What was the typical journey of a migrant once they arrived in mainland France? The activity of the Bumidom was divided into four categories: direct work placement, direct placement in training, placement after demobilization, family reunification. *Red arrow:* with qualifications (*building on the left:* recruitment). *Green arrow:* without qualifications (*building on the right:* training center). Bumidom had established its own vocational training centers for adults (FPA), also called "adaptation centers for metropolitan life." Men and women were assigned there differently: Simadres (69), Crouy-sur-Ourcq (77). Between 1962 and 1981, Bumidom's training centers saw 20,000 people pass through.

on the right panel we see this same woman in distress as she finds herself unable to prepare for the medical school entrance examination (*PN*, 161). Instead, she is stuck in a low-wage position (a nursing aide, when she wanted to become a doctor), and she is juggling a demanding job and the pressing responsibilities of domestic life (she is depicted holding a baby's bottle; her child is behind her and a seemingly controlling husband is holding her shoulders insistently, requesting attention). Everything keeps her away from achieving her original aspirations. Caring responsibilities confine her, like many others who left with the BUMIDOM, in a restrictive framework. The relegation of care work—tasks done in the service of others—to migrants from the overseas departments during those years is made further apparent at the bottom of that same page: women are assigned a set of stereotypes, including the tendency to be "patiente" (patient), "douce" (gentle), "travailleuse" (hard-working), "dévouée" (devoted), and "résiliente" (resilient), among others, that eventually constrains them to entering a caring role.

All these adjectives help underline that the work of care is undoubtedly defined by outward attention: paying attention to others and/or their environment, performing tasks that mobilize concern and attentiveness. These are adjectives that may be considered 'good' qualities to begin with but might all too often become an instrument of domination, a naturalized means to maintain an Antillean-specific pool of domestic workers.[12] Through its structural organization, the BUMIDOM therefore combines a social, gender, and racial organization of care work and the stereotyping of Antillean women to produce a hierarchy of attention, where the one who is required or expected to give attention receives very little, if not none. "Care is attention," Laugier suggests (2021, 65). For Laugier, the French substantive "attention" is the most adequate to capture the polysemy of the term "care" in English as she considers derivations of the word to define what she calls "le sujet du care" (the subject of caring). The subject of caring, according to Laugier, is "attentif" or "attentionné" (attentive), or "fait attention" (takes care) (2006, 360, 362). But because attention can be asymmetrical, it appears to be a double-edged sword—which Ega both denounces and seeks to overturn. For instance, Ega describes her encounter with Yolande, a woman she meets for the first time in tears at her neighborhood church. Yolande works as a live-in maid for a wealthy family in Marseille and describes to Ega the strenuous situation in which she finds herself. A lady ("une dame"; *LN*, 30), Yolande explains, paid for her to come to France and work at her service; Yolande makes 220 francs per month, but 150 go toward the reimbursement of her transatlantic travel, leaving her with 70 francs for herself and her two children living in Martinique (*LN*, 30).[13] As a carer, Yolande is vulnerable to abuse and exploitation—she has very limited means and mobility.

After this first encounter, Ega details the time when she went to the "villa [des] *maîtres* [de Yolande]" (the *masters'* villa, emphasis mine) only to find Yolande "un genou enveloppé d'une bande Velpeau, dans un jardin planté de laitues" (with her knee wrapped with an elastic bandage, standing in a lettuce garden) (*LN*, 36).[14] Ega transcribes the conversation that follows between her and Yolande:

> Yolande, aujourd'hui dimanche, que faites-vous avec cette bêche?
> —Je suis malade, j'ai des rhumatismes au genou, ils sont tous partis à la campagne.
> —Qui vous soigne donc?
> —Personne, j'ai acheté une pommade chez le pharmacien. *La dame a dit que* je n'ai pas encore droit à la Sécurité sociale. (*LN*, 36)
>
> Pourquoi faites-vous cela, puisque vous avez mal au genou?
> —*La dame a dit que* je suis bonne à tout faire! Je fais même le jardin!
> —Yolande, pourquoi ne venez-vous plus nous voir?

—*La dame a dit que* c'est depuis que je viens chez vous que je fais des manières. (*LN*, 37)

Yolande, today is Sunday, what are you doing with this spade?
—I'm unwell, I have rheumatism in the knee, all of them have gone to the countryside.
—Who is taking care of you then?
—Nobody. I bought some ointment at the pharmacy. *The lady said that* I can't register for social security yet.

Why are you doing this, since your knee is sore?
—*The lady said that* I am the maid! I even have to tend the garden!
—Yolande, why don't you come see us anymore?
—*The lady said that* I've been fussy since I started seeing you.

The repeated, almost automatic clause "La dame a dit que" ("the lady said that," the emphasis on this is mine) enacts the dispossession of Yolande's voice. Her responses to Ega's questions are invariably filtered through her employer's voice, guiding her every move and thought. As a live-in maid, Yolande is stripped of her right to move freely and decide for herself. This situation of "domination rapprochée" (or "close domination") to use French political scientist and sociologist Dominique Memmi's concept, reinforces the employer's control over domestic workers as well as supports an organized social isolation and lack of individual autonomy for the worker.

Memmi (2016) theorizes a situation of *close domination* to describe "une relation sociale plaçant ses protagonistes dans une situation d'interdépendance puissante, renforcée par le fait qu'ils se trouvent retenus de manière *quasi continue*, en situation de *coprésence physique*, dans un lieu *relativement unique et clos*" (a social relation positioning its protagonists in a situation of powerful interdependency, accentuated by the fact that they find themselves maintained quasi-continuously, in a situation of physical co-presence, in a place relatively unique and enclosed) (para. 1, emphases in original). In the context of domestic work as analyzed by Memmi, interdependency implies the existence of power hierarchies because the employer–worker relationship revolves around the worker's economic reliance and the employer's obscured dependence on the maintaining of their living space; the support bubble of those who appear "independent" is made invisible. Considering such a configuration, we thus see how networks of caring labor between the overseas departments and hexagonal France have been, from the beginning, placing workers in a precarious position, socially and economically. Curier, in fact, remarked that already at the "la Tour" training center in Crouy-sur-Ourcq women could feel quickly isolated socially and physically. Those who had relatives could visit them on the weekend and were able to rely on familial social support, but others "avaient l'autorisation d'aller se promener, sur la petite place du village" (were allowed to take a walk around the village square) (34). "C'était nos seules sorties. Ne connaissant pas les lieux, nous n'allions pas très loin" (These were our only excursions outside. Since we did not know the area, we would not go very far), Curier concluded.

Moreover, turning to the graphic narrative, we see that such a controlled and surveilled environment was maintained well after the newly trained maids were placed in a household. During their investigation, Oublié and Rousseau met with a certain "Mme X" (she asked to remain anonymous) who used to recruit all-female domestic staff through the BUMIDOM in the 1970s (Figure 2). The graphic narrative here incorporates reconstituted scenes from the past where hired domestic workers appear carrying out various tasks, such as cleaning, taking care of children, and answering the phone; in each panel, there is the lingering, disturbing presence of the employer(s) looking over the work being accomplished. For example, as a worker is shown answering the phone, her female employer stands over her shoulder smiling approvingly (*PN*, 179). In another instance, a domestic helper gives a juice box to a child while his parents stand at a distance seemingly pleased,

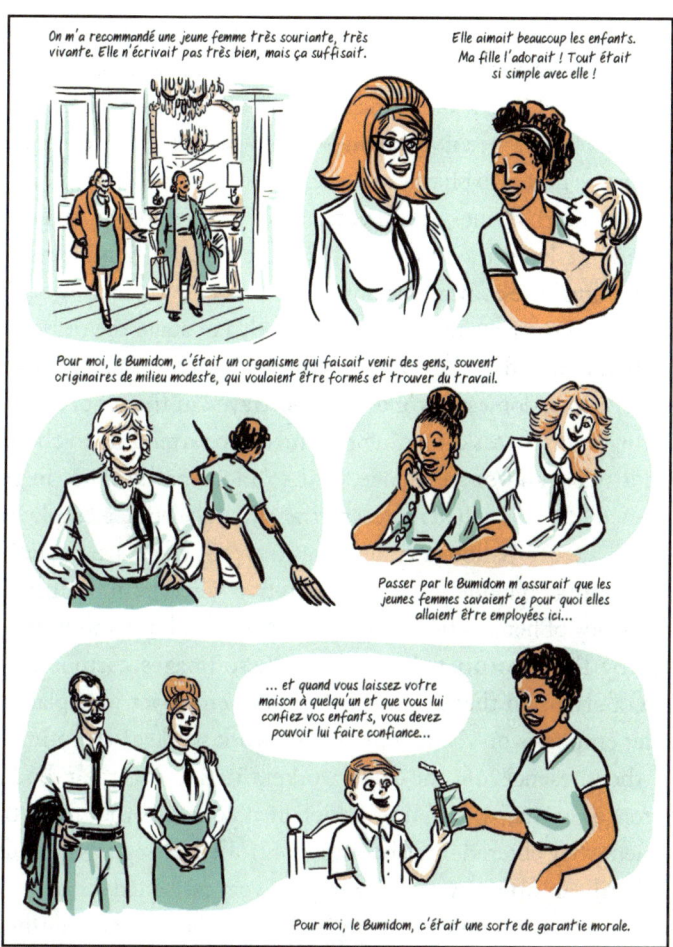

FIG. 2. *Péyi an nou*, page 179 © Steinkis, 2024

Text from left to right, in order of appearance:

I was recommended a very cheerful, lively woman. She didn't write very well, but it was enough. She really liked children. My daughter loved her. Everything was so easy with her. For me, the Bumidom was an organization that brought in people, often from modest backgrounds, who wanted to receive training and find work. Going through the Bumidom ensured that the young women knew what they were being hired for here . . . [*Speech bubble*] ". . . and when you entrust your home to someone and put your children in their care, you must be able to trust them . . ." For me, the Bumidom was a kind of moral guarantee.

as if touched by the apparent intimacy between their child and his carer. In one last example, the female employer is depicted in the foreground, while the domestic worker is seen from behind, holding a broom, her face not shown—the co-presence of worker and employer is linked explicitly and exclusively to the execution of the task (cleaning). Scenes of contentment caused by the appreciation of a task well-executed by the worker are visually significant not only to signal the continuous physical presence and scrutiny of the employer in the private workspace, but also to stage the degree of attention required of the domestic worker to satisfy their employer. On all counts, domestic workers are portrayed in the act of accomplishing a certain task, tending to someone or attending to chores, with a smile and/or in silence. Not so incidentally then, in the sequence of panels that represent the triptych worker-employer-task, no speech balloons appear, but instead, there are recitative passages that include Mme X's narrative voice, reinforcing the ascendancy of her position within the operational framework instituted by the BUMIDOM. For indeed, these images corroborate a form of attention that originates from the employer who places a strong emphasis on the completion of work while also diminishing the presence of the care worker, if not for their bodily existence on the page. All of which also confirms that from the moment they entered into the state-controlled caring labor industry, Antillean women were evolving in a very restricted framework, socially and economically marginalized—their voices muffled, their existence contained behind the doors of bourgeois households.

In effect, when Ega meets Yolande within the walls of her employers' mansion, she grapples with the immediate impact of a naturalized ascendancy within the social and racial organization of care work. Ega detects the woman's effacement as she obverses, "Yolande avait peur des gens, peur de son ombre, peur des Blancs, comme au plus beau temps de l'esclavage" (Yolande was afraid of people, afraid of her own reflection, afraid of white people, like in the days of slavery) (*LN*, 37). But Ega, unlike Yolande, retains her voice and integrity and chooses to use it first in defense of the woman she calls the "fille de [son] pays" (girl from her country) (*LN*, 36), and then for her to engage on the path to recovery of her own voice. Following her conversation with Yolande, Ega confronts "la dame" (the lady) insisting that her employee see a doctor for her knee pain. As *la dame* protests, Ega interferes to eventually announce Yolande's departure. In the end, "Yolande s'est vite habillée, et en clopinant elle m'a suivie; son visage rayonnait. Elle pouvait penser enfin que sa servitude prendrait fin" (Yolande dressed quickly, and followed me hobbling; her face was glowing with happiness. She might be thinking that her servitude would end) (*LN*, 38). Important in this exchange is the absence of first-person speech on the part of Yolande. In the dialogue section, Yolande's employer is in conversation with Ega, who literally speaks on behalf of the silent/silenced domestic worker.

Later, after Yolande has moved to Paris and is working as a hospital housekeeper, the narrative perspective momentarily shifts away from Ega's voice to bring into focus her own personal experience. Ega directly incorporates in the text the letter she received from Yolande; the third person ("The lady said that . . .") is replaced by the first person as the woman offers a nuanced and critical assessment of the working conditions specific to people coming from the French Caribbean, women in particular. "Il n'y a que des Antillaises qui font ce travail" (There are only Antillean women doing this work), Yolande remarks.[15] Yolande's letter is the narrative manifestation of her reclaimed presence, no longer filtered through the invasive and dominating voice of her employer ("The lady said that . . ."). Yet in her letter Yolande also alerts to the persistence of restraint and discretion on her part, as she describes an inability to speak out against an abusive accommodation situation for fear of being evicted. Unlike the two female "compatriotes" (compatriots) with whom Yolande rents a furnished room in Paris, she has never received a certificate of accommodation (*LN*, 89). Despite her precarious living situation, Yolande admits to Ega that "[elle] ne peu[t] rien y faire ni rien dire, c'est ainsi partout, et si [elle] le fai[t], [elle] risque d'être mise à la porte. . . . C'est dur mais c'est bien mieux que la dame à Marseille" (she cannot do or say anything, it is the same everywhere, and if she does, she risks being expelled. . . . It is hard but it is much better than with the lady in Marseille) (*LN*, 89). The opportunity to speak out more freely cedes here again to the seemingly inescapable social ascendancy of those who occupy positions of power relative to BUMIDOM workers, whether it be "la dame à Marseille" or "le patron du meublé"—positions from which they can easily assert control.

In a way, Ega disturbs the organization of such social relations from her position of close-distant observer-worker—a position from which she is able to penetrate an insidious system of oppression, assert her voice, and incorporate new forms of attention from within the structure of care work. How, then, does Ega remain close and distant, observer and worker at the same time? How does this twice dual position guarantee disruptive attention practices? Early on, Ega distinguishes her situation from that of her "sisters": she describes herself as a "cobaye volontaire" (voluntary experimental subject) (*LN*, 32), one who every night has a home to which she returns. To Carolina, she confesses, "je suis une privilégiée; quand je laisse madame et ses chiffons de poussière, j'ai un gîte, une famille qui m'attend et plus de travail que je n'ai de bras. . . . Comme je plains les Antillaises qui sont obligées de rester vingt-quatre heures avec ces lunatiques à qui elles servent de cobayes" (I am privileged; when I leave Madam and her dust rags, I have a house, a family waiting for me, and more work than I have arms for. . . . How sorry I feel for the Antillean women who are forced to stay twenty-four hours with these lunatics serving as their guinea pigs) (*LN*, 67).

Aware of social and racial hierarchy within the structure of care work, Ega amplifies her sense of home, turning the existence of a household into a salutary response to an alienating work experience. Quickly she gathers that, for Antillean women traveling to France in originally precarious conditions, work is predominantly exploitative and degrading. Is it that the house becomes Ega's "corner of the world, . . . [her] first universe, a real cosmos in every sense of the word" (Bachelard [1957] 2020, 32)?[16] Though, at first glance, the appraisal of the house we can find in Ega's *Lettres* appears somewhat removed from that of a place to peacefully dream and tuck oneself away. It is a space where she finds it difficult to proceed with her writing because she has her own "affaires intérieures" (private affairs) to deal with and is not always supported by her family, especially her husband who at first questions her literary ambition.

A housekeeper among "toutes les ménagères trop occupées" (all the other too busy housekeepers) (*LN*, 27), Ega mentions the routine household chores she diligently performs in her own home; her writing often happening in the early hours of the morning when nothing or no one will interrupt her work. Otherwise, she shows constant involvement in housework and childcare. "My little writer" is the nickname her husband has given her somewhat in mockery: "'Mon écrivain! Donne-moi mes chaussettes!' 'Mon écrivain, tu nous fais un gâteau?' Je lâche ma pointe Bic et je fais un gâteau. Mais quand il est parti, tôt le matin, et que mes supporters [her children] dorment encore, . . . je suis dans mon élément" ("My little writer! Give me my socks!" "My little writer, can you make us a cake?" I put my pen away, and I make a cake. But when he leaves, early in the morning, and my little supporters are still asleep, . . . I'm in my element) (*LN*, 35–36). Although Ega is working on her own project in her home space, her undivided attention is still expected to be primarily directed toward family caregiving and the completion of household chores. As we learn about what Ega accomplishes within the household and know very little about what her husband (often referred to by Ega as "mon mari," my husband, or "mon homme," my man) does, we might be tempted to assume that one form of care work is simply replaced by another as she moves from her work space to her home place. Why, then, does she consider herself to be in a privileged position? Would clinging to the idea of the home place as salvation be misleading?

In her essay "Homeplace: a site of resistance," bell hooks argues that for Black women globally to nurture a home in the midst of oppression and domination means to resist, restore dignity, and provide healing—it means "to include caring for one another, for children, for black men" (1990, 44). Although hooks speaks primarily of the legacies of the African American past, she confides the sense of shared history that she felt "reading about the plight of women domestic servants in South Africa, black women laboring in white homes" (43), similar to that which Ega feels toward Carolina when she reads about her daily struggle scavenging in the favela to keep herself and her children alive. For indeed, in the case of Ega, it appears that hearing another's voice speak up about oppression and women's struggles specifically had a liberating effect on her own, triggering a chain reaction of empowerment.

In hooks's argument about women's empowerment through homemaking in defiance of oppressive systems, she finds that "this task of making a homeplace, of making home a community of resistance, has been shared by Black women globally, especially Black women in white supremacist societies" (1990, 42). In effect, the homeplace, which Ega grows in large part, is what shields her away from a degrading and dehumanizing work environment. It may not be the restful (i.e., quiet) abode imagined by French philosopher Gaston Bachelard, but Ega's homeplace is nevertheless what helps her resist physical and psychological exploitation outside her home. As Ega observes, "J'arrive facilement à secouer le joug moral que comporte ce sacré métier parce que j'ai un toit, une famille à moi. Mais comme je comprends ces filles liées nuit et jour au service de ces sacrées dames" (I manage eventually to shake off the psychological yoke of that hell of a job because I have a home and a family of my own. But how I understand these girls bound to be in the service of those hellish women day and night) (*LN*, 193). What I am suggesting here is not that we overlook the seemingly disproportionate amount of care work (cleaning her own house, taking care of her children, or mending her husband's socks, for example) Ega executes within her own household, but that we equally acknowledge that it is the existence of a space outside of work, a homeplace to return to, that allows Ega's inner voice to resound throughout the text.

Reaping the fruits of her attentive homemaking, Ega finds within her homeplace the means to emancipate herself from the condition of domestic worker, to leave behind a world of alienating work through the transformative power of the homeplace and the encouragement and support she finds within it. Through recognition of who she is outside of the domestic work she performs in other people's homes, Ega is not subject to devaluation inside the home; rather, her children give importance to her dedication to writing, paying enthusiastic attention to her progress. "J'ai un public attentif qui me demande la suite de mon livre: mes enfants!" (I have an attentive audience who ask what happens next in my book: my children!) Ega announces to Carolina. "Ils me lisent! Ils rient! Ils s'exclament!" (They read my work! They laugh! They shout!) (*LN*, 50). The back-and-forth between the workplace, shaped by racial oppression and domination, and the homeplace, where her sense of integrity may be restored, is what challenges the trope of invisibility. Laugier reminds us, "What defines [good] care as work well done [is] discretion. And this discretion is the source of its devaluation" (2021, 75). As such, the tools of oppression are already scripted within the operative model of care work: the attention is thenceforth taken away from the caregiver, or care worker, to be placed on the executed task(s) and those benefiting from it. This model, promoted by the BUMIDOM, supports hierarchies of attention and truly helps consolidate the pernicious dynamics of race, gender, and class power.

Ega's inner voice is one that challenges the hierarchical structure of care work by recentering initially a self-regarding first-person. As she describes her search to be hired as a housekeeper, Ega is resolved to find a position that she finds suitable, having regard for her own personal obligations. She explains,

> Gentiment la placeuse m'a demandé si je ne pouvais pas me libérer toute la journée, j'aurais le repas de midi compris dans mes gages. Puisque je cuisine à outrance pour ma marmaille, le repas des autres ne m'intéresse pas. Et puis il me faut au moins

une demi-journée pour m'occuper de ma propre maison, je refusai donc. (*LN*, 127)

The employment agent kindly asked if I could make myself available for the whole day, my lunch would be paid. Since I cook an excessive amount of food for my children, I had no interest for other people's meals. Moreover, I need at least a half-day to look after my own house. I therefore turned down her offer.

Her exercise of self-regard is to set limits and boundaries for the workplace, giving importance to that other space: the home she nurtures for herself and her family. The idea of a personal threshold plays an important role in questioning what is usually expected, if not demanded, of Antillean women in need of work, in particular in the case of live-in maids. Unlike many others, Ega retains the ability to choose, which contrapuntally serves to heighten the extensive carelessness toward caregivers, working within the interplay of care work and organized migration from French overseas departments at the time.

Juxtaposing Ega's inner voice against the relationship between employer and Antillean domestic workers, the dynamic of domination and subjugation so far operating behind the closed doors of bourgeois mansions is made apparent. Through Ega's narrative intervention, attention shifts to those who suffer neglect and abuse. In part, her narrative voice is one that fosters dissent and resistance on her sole behalf. One example that highlights that purpose is when Ega reclaims her individuality against an employer's tendency to anonymize domestic staff. "C'est clair et net. Qu'on m'appelle Renée et je répondrai quand je penserai qu'il s'agit de moi" (I'm saying it loud and clear. If they call me "Renée," I will only answer when I think they're asking for me) (*LN*, 175). Renée is the woman Ega agreed to replace after learning that, although Renée had been suffering from abdominal pain for three months, her employer suggested ("Madame a dit que . . ." (Madam said that . . .)

(*LN*, 174) Renée only get her operation after she reimbursed the 90,000 francs she had "borrowed" to come work in the Hexagon. Here Ega emphasizes a conscious decision to challenge the employer's assumption of the interchangeability of domestic workers. Ega's narrative voice above all achieves a more dramatic shift of attention as Ega's first-person inner voice becomes exteriorized initially through an intimate one-way correspondence with Carolina, and then through the publication of *Lettres* posthumously. Ega's imagined epistolary exchange first creates the possibility for attention to be deployed to self and others, and second supports, via the position of exteriority of the written text, the expansion of practices of attentive looking to lives that have largely been sidelined.

The undertaking of incorporating voice, of shedding light on individuals who tell about the not-so-distant but largely unspoken historical episode of the BUMIDOM is taken up by Jessica Oublié and Marie-Ange Rousseau in the graphic narrative *Péyi an nou* (2017). This chapter previously analyzed passages of this graphic narrative in relation to care work, and this last section focuses on the formal properties of the medium to constitute a BUMIDOM-specific archive of voices made visible and taking up space on the page. Against the silences around the BUMIDOM—which, through the lens of care work, appear to be somewhat by design—*Péyi an nou* expands the form of individual expression while also pointing out a largely shrouded historical context. The authors make clear that this work is their initial dive into a chapter of French history that had been completely unknown to them and others.

A random internet search fortuitously served as Oublié's point of departure as she prepared for a trip to Guadeloupe to visit her family in 2015. Leaving with the original intent to write her family history under the project title "Restore the Story," Oublié stumbled upon the name of the state agency, which later caused an uproar at the dinner table with her relatives in Guadeloupe. Amid a heated discussion about the contentious prospect of leaving the island to find work in the Hexagon, Uncle Albert exclaimed, in disjointed speech over three consecutive panels, "Les enfants . . . Tout ce que vous devez savoir . . . si vous êtes nés en France . . . c'est la faute du BUMIDOM!" (Kids . . . All you need to know . . . if you were born in France . . . it's BUMIDOM's fault!) (*PN*, 12). These were the words that prompted Oublié to explore further a past about which she knew nothing, starting with an investigation into the extent of Afro-Caribbean-descended people's knowledge of the history of the overseas departments—or the lack thereof.

As she returns to Paris, Oublié is portrayed in a sequence of phone exchanges with close friends and family members living in the Hexagon who have familial ties to the French Caribbean; she asks them about their own relationship to these territories (especially Guadeloupe and Martinique) (*PN*, 14–15). Some admit that they only consider the islands to be their parents' birthplace; others mention their perceived cultural status as *métros* (or *métropolitains*, Metropolitans), which immediately lays bare a marked difference between those who live in the French Antilles and those born in the Hexagon.[17] At the conclusion of this inquiry, Kelly, Oublié's sister, observes, "Je trouve qu'il y a un vrai manque de représentation de notre culture et notre histoire dans la société française" (I think our culture and history is clearly underrepresented within French society at large) (*PN*, 15).

Péyi an nou then creates the possibility to imagine beyond the ignorance of or indifference to the past of the overseas departments through the medium of graphic narrative.[18] "What kind of visual-verbal literacy can respond to the needs of the present moment?" asked Marianne Hirsch (2004, 1212), a question Hillary Chute aptly borrows to explore the ethical considerations of representations of history in the graphic narrative form (2008, 462). This question also readily applies to our inquiry into the possibility of forefronting the BUMIDOM experience in the arrangement of visual and verbal elements. In *Péyi an nou*, this means promoting modes of disruption of a hierarchy of attention made most visible through the lens of a BUMIDOM-specific labor pool of carers. For indeed, the graphic narrative expresses Oublié's urgency to show and tell the invisibilized history of the BUMIDOM. How to, in other words, reverse the mechanisms of inattention, of uncaring, deeply rooted in the structure of the BUMIDOM? The composition of the graphic narrative, in fact, lends itself to an inversion in practices of attention designed for the perpetuation of privilege and power over minoritized populations. Early on in *Péyi an nou*, the reliance on gathering and conveying audible and visual testimonies is made clear by incorporating depictions of the recording devices such as voice recorders and the instances where Oublié and/or Rousseau are seen taking notes. A combined visibility and audibility means that the reader sees on the page the conversations and reconstituted dialogues between the author(s) (Oublié occasionally conducts interviews on her own and records content on a voice recorder) and the scholars or individuals who left through the BUMIDOM. In this context, the distribution of verbality (i.e., words transcribed from testimonies or archival documents) and the organization of physical presence indicates an active manipulation of visual-verbal form to the purpose of increasing and valorizing minoritized voices—a practice that closely aligns with Ega's dialogic approach to storytelling.[19]

To further explore the specificity of the comic form, critic Ann Miller (2007) writes in her groundbreaking study of French comic art that there are five types of text identifiable in *bande dessinée*, among which are the narrative voice-over or *récitatif* and the dialogue, both which are of interest to us here. Miller proposes that the récitatif signals a more (or less) assertive narrative voice; when it is used discreetly, it is "usually separated from the pictorial space by a box which adheres to the top of the frame"; sometimes, though, it may appear with no box, "indicating, perhaps, an absence of narrative distance from the events portrayed" (2009, 97). Here the possibility of disruption of such formal features is highlighted when Miller mentions briefly that manipulating the récitatif may more or less assert the narrating voice. Thus, disordering these formal codes can concretize a geography of caring, the possibility for attention being created in the layout of the visually and verbally reconstituted testimonies.

The interview setting, in effect, perfectly illustrates an attention-making process relying on active listening. The practice of listening that takes place in *Péyi an nou* is more than just hearing, or in this case reading, what a person is expressing; it also makes space available for other voices to emerge, alternating with that of the authors and building an expansive archive of the BUMIDOM. Such practice is one that is made possible through the erosion of the formal textual and visual characteristics that Miller distinguishes between the récitatif (usually delineated by a box) and the dialogue (in speech balloons). Rather than a "blurring between the narratorial voice and the voice of the characters" in an interview setting (Wimbush 2018, 21), the voices of the interviewees telling their stories, I argue, progressively overtake the voices of the authors.

One aspect of this swap of primary narrative voice takes effect when the authorial voice gradually diminishes from framed récitatif to speech balloon within the frame when, for example, Oublié and Rousseau are portrayed conducting a phone interview with a certain Édouard, who left Martinique for the Hexagon in 1962 at the age of twenty-two (Figure 3). Édouard, who had since then returned to the island, calls them from his home in Rivière Salée. As the phone conversation opens, two frames are juxtaposed on the panel depicting the location of Oublié and Rousseau in Paris on the left-hand side and Édouard in Rivière Salée on the right-hand side. The next frame shows only the interviewee sitting in his living room. Two types of text coexist here: the récitatif, which signals the authors' narrative voice and situates how they have come into contact with Édouard (a call for testimonies circulated on Facebook), and the dialogue, enclosed in a speech balloon, which foregrounds the voice of Édouard, the primary visible speaker during the conversation. For indeed, Oublié and Rousseau play a minor role in this interview sequence to focus attention on

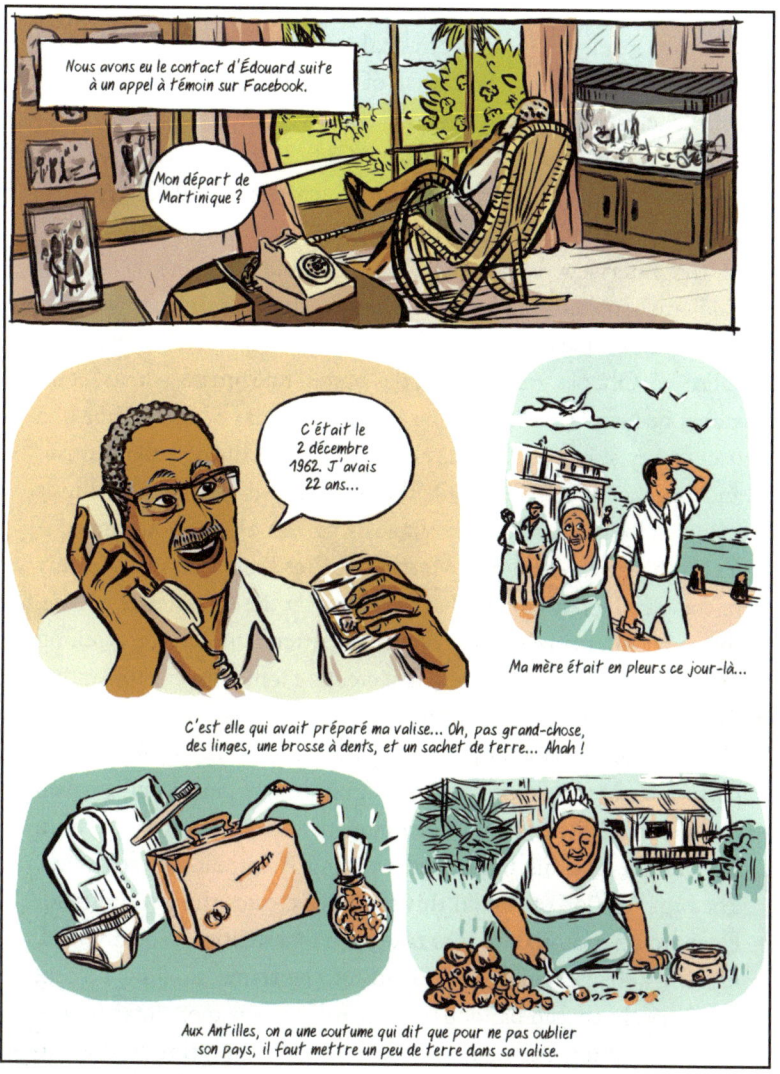

FIG. 3. *Péyi an nou*, page 66 © Steinkis, 2024

Text from left to right, in order of appearance:

We got in touch with Édouard following a witness call on Facebook. [*Speech bubble*] "My departure from Martinique?" [*Speech bubble*] "It was December 2, 1962. I was 22 years old . . ." My mother was in tears that day . . . She was the one who packed my suitcase . . . Oh, not much, some clothes, a toothbrush, and a small pouch of soil . . . Ahah! In the Caribbean, we have a tradition that says to avoid forgetting your country, you must put a bit of soil in your suitcase.

Édouard's voice; Oublié's physical presence only reappears in a couple of frames over the course of the seven-panel segment, her voice enclosed in speech balloons within the frame (*PN*, 68, 70). Except for these two instances, Oublié and Rousseau are not depicted, thus symbolically neither seen nor heard. Even their questions are omitted from the dialogue; rather, their participation in the interview is conveyed through the combined effect of Édouard's spoken reactions and ellipses. He says, for example, "Ma mère était en pleurs ce jour-là. . . . C'est elle qui avait préparé ma valise . . . Oh, pas grand chose, des linges, une brosse à dents, et un sachet de terre" (My mother was in tears the day I left. . . . She had packed my suitcase. . . . Oh, not much, some linen, a toothbrush, and a packet of soil) (*PN*, 66). The three dots indicating the ellipsis followed by Édouard's reply suggests he was asked about the content of his suitcase leaving Martinique. Yet the distribution of text in the panel strives to emphasize primarily the interviewee's voice, the so far minoritized story. Moreover, after Édouard starts telling his story, the frames are unboxed, creating a narrative whole rather than freezing each moment in the story, singling them out. Here also the speech balloon is making way for a récitatif whose first-person narrator becomes Édouard himself, who, in an undisturbed manner, reminisces about the circumstances of his departure from Martinique and his living and working situation over the years. The organization of text in this sequence creates the possibility for Édouard's narratorial voice to take over, for attention to be diverted. His story then expands the bounds of the frame: no longer a text contained in speech balloons, Édouard's story is momentarily centered, becoming the main narrative thread, the primary voice to which we pay attention. Instead of a focus on his full name or personal details—which would run the risk of making a witness traceable who may have wished to remain anonymous—the emphasis is, here and throughout, on the treatment of voices so far unheard, from which the power of attention is derived, along with the possibility to reverse the silence around the BUMIDOM.

In another interview sequence, attention is again textually and visually achieved within the curated space of the graphic narrative but is also staged expanding outward, extending beyond the scene represented. The endeavor to create an archive of voices, as pursued throughout *Péyi an nou*, reaches apotheosis in the formulation of a far-reaching form of attention. How can attention then be extended beyond the time and space in which the story is told to assist in the archive-making enterprise? The continual visual presence of the voice recorder, which Oublié diligently carries with her during interviews, becomes the metonymic evidence of the construction of the archive, therefore constituting an outward-reaching supplement to an internally formed attention. The sequence that follows incorporates visual-textual devices of attention, which when combined operate from within the graphic narrative while also containing an indication of an exteriority.

For this interview, Oublié visits Léo, a friend of her grandparents, who lives in Le Gosier, Guadeloupe (Figure 4). An encounter there with a group of his friends is represented; they have all gone through the BUMIDOM, either for work or for family reunification (starting in the 1970s). The close-up on the voice recorder (*PN*, 112) marks the beginning of a staged interview during which Oublié's presence is again rendered marginal. In one scene in particular, four elderly individuals (Gilda, Suzy, Martial, and Léo) are portrayed reminiscing about their past lives in Paris, building on each other's memories and, more importantly, with no mediation from Oublié (*PN*, 115). Again, the conversation eclipses the boundaries of the frame; Oublié is depicted to the side holding the voice recorder while a swirling of speech balloons releases the voices of first-hand witnesses, making it possible to center their migration experiences, "les bons et les mauvais moments" (good and bad times), equally.

Thus, over the course of the several interviews conducted by either Oublié and Rousseau together or Oublié on her own, the authors may appear verbally marginal, but they remain visually

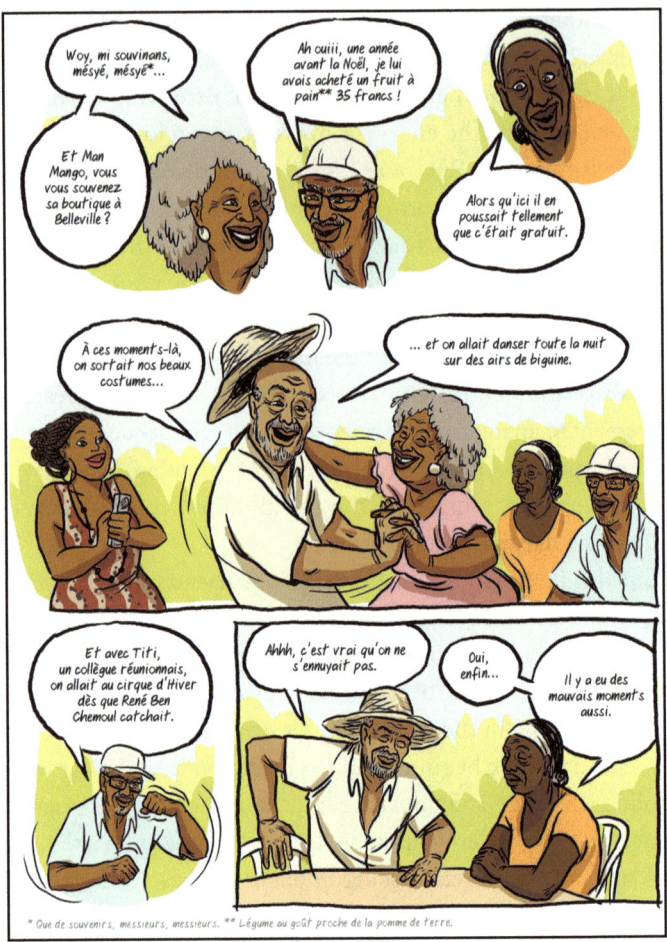

FIG. 4. *Péyi an nou*, page 115 © Steinkis, 2024

Text from left to right, in order in which the speech bubbles appear:

"So many memories, gentlemen, gentlemen." "And Man Mango, do you remember her shop in Belleville?" "Ah yes! A year before Christmas, I had bought a breadfruit from her for 35 francs!" "Whereas here, they grew so abundantly that they were free." "During those times, we would take out our finest suits . . ." ". . . and dance all night to the sounds of the beguine." "And with Titi, a colleague from Reunion, we would go to the Cirque d'Hiver whenever René Ben Chemoul was wrestling." "Ahhh, it's true that we always had something to do." "Yes, well . . ." "There were some bad times too."

present and so does the recording device. The consistent visual presence of the voice recorder in fact metonymically inaugurates voices made accessible, securing transmission and audibility across the spaces and times spanning the graphic narrative. Within *Péyi an nou*, the hypervisibility of the object, which sometimes appears alone in a frame, contributes to the creation of a listening ecosystem, one that initially fosters and maintains listening within the graphic narrative and which eventually makes us see the possibility of reversing the unheard, unseen, and undervalued incorporated within the BUMIDOM through an attentive listening practice. By tracing the presence of the object throughout, the listening ecosystem embedded within the narrative is revealed. When Oublié, for instance, meets with historian Monique Milia-Marie-Luce from the Université des Antilles to learn about the history of the now overseas departments, Rousseau is absent, but the information is shown being recorded, testifying to its subsequent transportability and accessibility. In fact, as Oublié concludes her interview with Milia-Marie-Luce, the last frame of the sequence includes a close-up of the voice recorder she holds in her hand (*PN*, 32).

In the following frame, the voice recorder has traveled to a new location; it is now sitting on a table in Oublié's apartment and again appears in close-up as it plays Milia-Marie-Luce's *exposé* to Rousseau, who exudes confusion: "Oh là là, ça a l'air assez compliqué tout ça" (Oh là là, it all seems quite complex), Rousseau exclaims (*PN*, 33). The graphic narrative makes visible the fact that the 'discovery' of the previously unknown migration may first result in bewilderment and apprehension, which is crucial here. It establishes that the sudden cognizance of the BUMIDOM and how it has affected people's lives is paradoxically met with a just as sudden awareness of a pending burden of attention, or what French philosopher Simone Weil calls "un effort d'attention" (an effort of attention) (1966, 68). Weil describes this effort as the suspension of thought, allowing the mind to remain available and receptive as one turns toward another individual. The suspension of thought, Weil proposes, leaves us "disponible, vide et pénétrable à l'objet" (detached, empty, and ready to be penetrated by the object) (1966, 72).[20] Such a disposition may be one to seek to reach through the process of becoming available and open to the reality of other people, to the stories of others. Oublié and Rousseau's grappling with the realities of emigration from the French Caribbean might well introduce readers to this process. Although the object of transmission (the voice recorder) becomes the archiving tool that assists the authors in the visual and verbal composition of witnesses, the active work of care contained in the effort of attention still falls to individuals like Oublié and Rousseau. The development of the faculty of attention that we see taking shape in the graphic narrative is thus what maintains the conversation and the circulation and continuity of these stories.

I now repeat my previous question: How can attention be extended beyond the time and space in which the story is told? What I am suggesting in the end is that the practice of attention acquired within the graphic narrative, starting with Oublié and Rousseau, is propelled toward the outside of the story world. The closing scene of *Péyi an nou* takes place at a bookstore in Paris where the two authors are attending the signing by Pap Ndiaye (Figure 5) of his essay *La condition Noire: Essai sur une minorité française* (The Black condition: essay on a French minority; 2008). In this work, Ndiaye analyzes issues of racism, citizenship, and national identity in France against the background of the history of Black people. In particular, Ndiaye discusses the question of intersectional in/visibility in contemporary France, and he eventually concludes, "Il reste maintenant à . . . écrire les bouts manquants de notre histoire collective" (Now we have to write the missing parts of our collective history) (2008, 205). In the last frame, Ndiaye is holding a printed copy of *Péyi an nou*—through which the effort of attention toward minoritized voices and histories has been initiated. In turn, Oublié and Rousseau, appearing in profile, are turning one eye to the readers, inviting us to continue this attention. As evidence of the potential response to this call for attention, it is notable that several panels from *Péyi an nou*

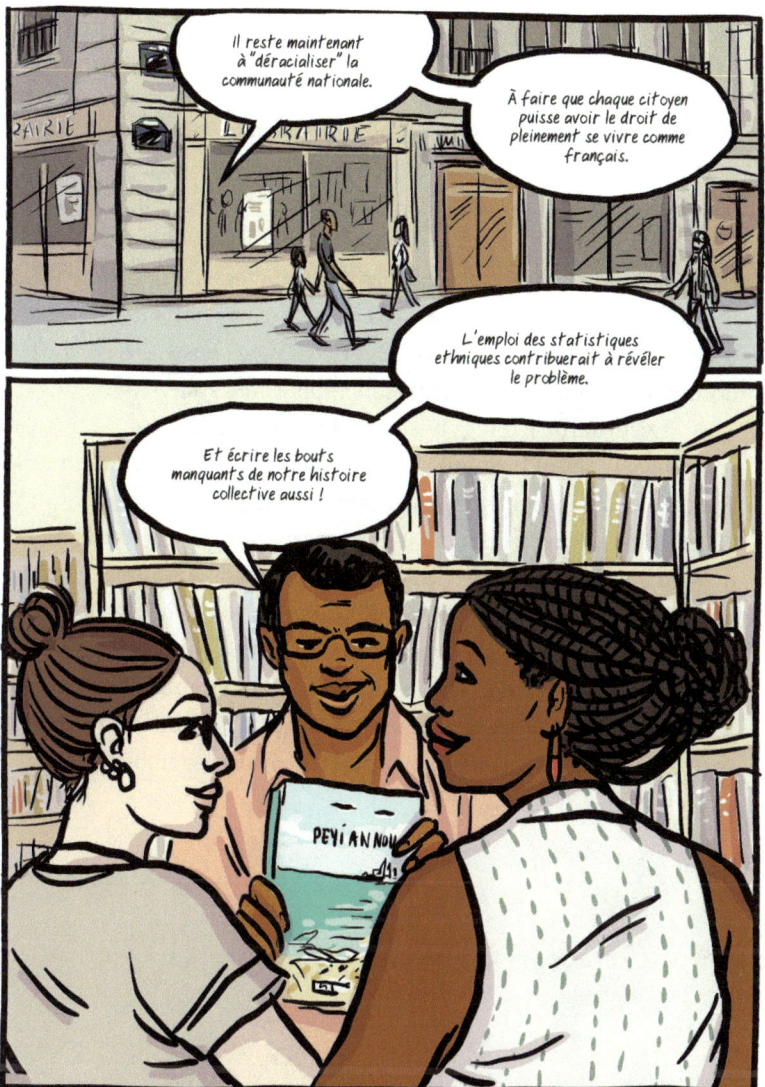

FIG. 5. *Péyi an nou*, page 205 © Steinkis, 2024

Text from left to right, in order in which the speech bubbles appear: "We now face the task of 'deracializing' the national community." "Of ensuring that every citizen has the right to fully live as French." "The use of ethnic statistics would help shed light on the problem." "And write the missing pieces of our collective history as well!"

have been included in the permanent collection of the Musée National de l'Histoire de l'Immigration in Paris since 2019.

The line of continuity from Ega to Oublié and Rousseau is found in the creation and perpetuation of a practice of visibility, a renewed effort of attention toward minoritized lives. Through the particular intersection of caring labor and the BUMIDOM, we see the deep entanglement of the state agency with the increase, if not the making, of invisibility for those tasked to care, to pay attention to others' needs. As a clandestine writer, Ega chose the path of domestic service to document a state-sponsored system of oppression. Eventually having been published, her *Lettres* find an addressee, if not in Carolina, in us, allowing these shrouded experiences of domesticity to move from silence into ownership of voice. By speaking from her own perspective, Ega, as "aquela que diz não à sombra" (the one who denies her shadow) (Siqueira and de Castilhos Lucena 2020, 57), calls attention to the impact of the generalized carelessness toward those groomed to care. She also highlights a path toward the necessary work of attention that such a legacy convokes. This call, which is taken up by Oublié and Rousseau through *Péyi an nou*, may ultimately be extended beyond the story world.

3
Inhabiting the Land after Environmental Damage

In a gender-focused analysis of literary representations of the Caribbean landscape, French scholars Natacha d'Orlando, Cécile Chapon, and Marine Cellier (2020) open their discussion of texts by Gisèle Pineau and Jamaica Kincaid with a necessarily unambiguous quote about the fundamental interaction between the living environment and human activities from Guadeloupean writer Daniel Maximin's *Les fruits du cyclone* (2006): "La nature dans la Caraïbe n'est pas un décor, c'est un personnage central de son histoire" (In the Caribbean, nature is not a setting, it is a central character in its history) (81). For indeed, as Édouard Glissant reminds us in *Le discours antillais*, "Notre paysage est son propre monument. La trace qu'il signifie est repérable par-dessous. C'est tout histoire" ("Our landscape is its own monument: its meaning can only be traced on the underside. It is all history") ([1981] 1997, 32; 1989, 11); the Caribbean landscape bears the marks of human history, in particular of the violence of the Middle Passage and of the colonial extractivist relationship to the human and nonhuman worlds it encompasses. As regards the engagement with both the landscapes of the region and the historical human activities that have shaped it, Elizabeth DeLoughrey, Renée Gosson, and George Handley highlight, in their introduction to *Caribbean*

Literature and the Environment (2005), the difficulty for writers to address these two aspects simultaneously. They note, in particular, the tenuous negotiation between the colonial history of environmental degradation of the region and the drive to retrieve what has been lost. The risk, however, is of turning to tropes of exoticism rooted in colonial imagination, such as the formulation of the "natural" world as "the site of Europe's lost Eden" (Burns 2008, 20).[1] Literature plays, in any case, a crucial role in mediating the complex historical entanglements of people and place while thinking through ways for the self and others to inhabit the world with the knowledge of that past as well as imagining sustainable futures. The literary manipulations of a traumatic, wounded Caribbean landscape—one that has been violently removed from an Eden, which is "your home, the place you are from" (Kincaid 2020)—can very much lay out for us the terms of caring imaginaries in the present, calling out the effect of long-lasting carelessness while contributing to our experimental futures.

In this chapter I am particularly interested in looking at literary representations and negotiations of the Caribbean landscape as a site dramatically altered by "colonial inhabitation" (or "l'habiter colonial" as defined by Malcolm Ferdinand in *Une écologie décoloniale*, 2019), as well as at the reimaginings of human relationships to that landscape.[2] How does the literary negotiate the tension between the inescapability of colonial damage and the possibility of recovery? As such, I situate my exploration of literary representations of the Caribbean landscape and care at the intersection of two attitudes that might appear contradictory at first: one of removal from and another of groundedness in a world damaged by colonial appropriation, exploitation, and extraction. Once set in tension, or rather alongside each other, these two attitudes contain a proposition for expansive and lucid caring imaginaries—expansive in the sense that they consider the human and nonhuman worlds in their interconnectedness, and lucid in the sense that they assume an awareness of the environmental and human legacies of colonialism. This chapter, then, examines literary vegetal-human imaginaries centered around contrasting formulations of the garden.

I first discuss the novel *Morne Câpresse* by Gisèle Pineau (2008), where the reader meets the Congrégation des Filles de Cham (the Congregation of the Daughters of Cham), a self-enclosed community of women formed by Sainte Mère Pacôme, a former RATP agent turned spiritual guide.[3] They live on top of a morne[4]—the emblematic historic site of Maroon resistance—and live off subsistence gardening away from the devastated "world below" ("le monde d'en bas"—the expression is used throughout the novel).

Second, I consider *Tropiques toxiques* (2020) by Jessica Oublié (scenarist), Nicola Gobbi (illustrator), Kathrine Avraam (photographer), and Vinciane Lebrun (colorist). I investigate how the usage of chlordecone, a toxic and persistent insecticide used to eradicate banana weevils in the French Caribbean between the years 1972 and 1993, and its adverse effect on human and nonhuman health as well as the living environment are mediated through the medium of graphic narrative. In this regard, we see, for example, that one of the many harmful consequences of this generalized contamination is the brutal interruption of traditional sustenance garden practices—the Creole garden or *jardin créole*.

How, then, can these aesthetics and ethics of the garden in their compromised forms over time act as a template for caring for the environment as well as for caring relations between the human and nonhuman worlds? How are they each, respectively, an indication of what it means to turn our attention to a world marked by a history of colonial spoliation and devastation? And finally, what emerges from their being compromised in different ways over time?

"Vous pouvez m'appeler Sœur Lucia" (You can call me Sister Lucia) (11)—Soeur Lucia, one of the most established members of the Congrégation des Filles de Cham founded by the self-proclaimed Sainte Mère Pacôme, opens Gisèle Pineau's novel *Morne Câpresse* (2008; hereafter *MC*) with an address to a "you" unidentified at first. Line is the young woman introduced to the Congrégation as she searches for her missing little sister Mylène, but the "you" in the opening address may generally refer to anyone (Line's name only appears in the last paragraph of that chapter) who has come to the morne to heal and repair, at least initially. For indeed, Pacôme, having left behind a bleak existence in hexagonal France working as a RATP agent, has returned to her native Guadeloupe on a mission she believes was entrusted to her by the spirit of the ancestors, the voices of the former enslaved. Pacôme first sets to searching for her unknown relatives—the numerous children born to Charles Débaury, her absent father, an inveterate seducer; then she sets to rescuing "les filles égarées du pays" (the country's lost girls), "les sauver de tous les Charles Débaury.... Et puis sauver la Guadeloupe.... Sauver le monde" (saving them from all the Charles Débaurys . . . and finally saving Guadeloupe . . . is saving the world) (*MC*, 21). Defined as such, Pacôme's rescue mission is linked to the reappropriation of a foundational narrative because the primary condition for the formation of the Congrégation is to reassemble an original filiation. For indeed, the character first tasks herself with locating the dispersed children of her father Charles Débaury, piecing together a missing linear genealogy. But she then aims to rescue "les filles égarées du pays [Guadeloupe]"—all of whom form the foundation of Pacôme's aspiring women-only community, an alternative version of family. Following Pacôme, saving women from patriarchal oppression by re-embedding them in a seemingly restored nature may thus have the potential to formulate another way of inhabiting the world.

Considering the initial motivations driving the creation of this women-exclusive community, it might seem evident that the Congrégation represents a significant step toward revitalization of both women and the habitats greatly impacted by colonial inhabitation. Originally the Congrégation appears to be a deliberate effort to counterbalance an abusive and destructive way of inhabiting the world, one that is anchored historically in the exploitation of human and nonhuman lives and environmental destruction.

More specifically, in tying together the denunciation of environmental devastation and forms of patriarchal oppression, such as the abusive behavior of a husband or a father ("[les] coups d'un mari, [les] dérives d'un père" [the blows of a husband, the abuses of a father]; *MC*, 30) in the depiction of Guadeloupe at the turn of the twenty-first century, Pacôme's women-only Congrégation takes shape as a reaction to the persistent violent ways of inhabiting the world specific to the legacy of colonial rule. More to the point, Pineau's fiction spells out for each woman joining the ranks of the Congrégation the joint legacy of the exploitation and abuse of racialized and gendered bodies, the dispossession and degradation of the land, and the squandering of resources (Ferdinand 2019, 2022; Glissant [1981] 1997; Sheller 2003). And there is also, conversely, the promise of radicality that lies, at least at first glance, in the possibility of another place that is not here, one that would be "pre-industrial; pre-colonial" or even "pré-plantationnaire" (pre-plantation), to borrow the words of Natacha d'Orlando et al. (2020, 9). The Congrégation is, in effect, built on hopes of reappropriation—the community has settled on a former coffee plantation 'gifted' by a *béké*—of self-reliance—Soeur Lucia affirms that they live on "bonnes terres" (good lands) that provide "le manger de chaque jour" (food every day) (*MC*, 27)—and of healing for both women and the land they inhabit. "How can we obtain the land, and bread to eat?" Frantz Fanon asks (1966, 52). Presented as a restored bountiful paradise, Pacôme's community may well appear like the long-awaited refuge away from the racial, gender, and environmental violence enveloping the world the Daughters of Cham have just left behind.

In this regard alone, when Line concludes her climb to reach Morne Câpresse, her eyes meet idyllic vegetation, a vision of peaceful bliss that is quite evocative of "[l]es peintures haïtiennes où le jardin d'Eden est représenté sur cette terre, paré de tous les arbres de la Création donnant des fruits à profusion" (Haitian paintings where the Garden of Eden is represented on this Earth, dressed with the trees of Creation abundantly yielding fruit) (*MC*, 58).[5]

"Les plantations étaient amoureusement soignées, ordonnées, tracées au cordeau" (plantations were groomed with love, ordered, trimmed in a straight line), Line continues to describe (*MC*, 58). In reference to the organization of the plantation, the adverb "amoureusement" (or "with love") already points to the rewriting of the plantation not as a site of violence but rather as a space allowing for peaceful and good-hearted cultivation practices. It is a space the women of the Congrégation industriously tend to but that they appear to have reclaimed as well, at least in theory. And so Mère Pacôme's alternative society seemingly addresses the plight of marginalized and suffering women, offering them a reprieve from their reported state of neglect and disempowerment in urban settings. The narrator observes that before joining the Congrégation they were "femelles zombies des villes" (city female zombies) (*MC*, 31), as if they had lost both their bodies and their individual consciousness. Additionally, the establishment of the Congrégation also appears to support environmental restoration in the face of an ecological peril linked to former plantations that have fallen into disrepair.

Imagined as the site of reparation against a failing reality, Mère Pacôme's Congrégation attests, at the level of conception, to the anticolonial ecofeminist nature of her vision. The Congrégation, indeed, reacts to the abuse of both women and nature (Griffin 1978; Merchant 1980; Mies and Shiva 1993; Salleh 1997) in contemporary French Caribbean society, while integrating the legacy of colonial slavery and economy of extraction.[6] That said, although the Congrégation envisions a profound reimagining of its surroundings, fostering caring human interaction with the environment while providing a sanctuary for women, there is trouble afoot. What then has gone wrong, I dare ask? For over the course of Line's incursion into the community of women in search of her missing sister, the novel chronicles the rise and ultimate fall of the Congrégation. Here, I am particularly interested in retracing Line's steps as she evolves through this "copie du Paradis" (imitation of Paradise) (*MC*, 162), examining the Congrégation as a template for "*une guérison manquée*" or a slip in the act of healing, in the act of caring for these distraught human lives in a ravaged landscape. For indeed, Sainte Mère Pacôme believes she is meeting the needs of the women of the Congrégation by providing and maintaining "un endroit idéal à l'abri des tentations, de la perdition" (an ideal place away from temptation and vice) (*MC*, 89). And yet, why can Pacôme's project only ever be an "imitation of Paradise"? Why has the endeavor to rescue afflicted women paired with the restoration of an unspoiled place—which, let us not forget, has been witness to the colonial plundering of resources—turned out to be profoundly deceptive?

The multiple scholars who have proposed their readings of *Morne Câpresse* stress the concerns and limitations of Pacôme's utopian aspirations by calling attention to the behind-the-scenes presence of a not-so-charming *locus amoenus*. Antje Ziethen, for instance, makes mention of a "Paradis [qui] s'effrite" (crumbling Paradise) (2012, 59); Natacha d'Orlando and Tina Harpin call the Daughters of Cham's garden "un leurre d'hétérotopie heureuse" (a deceitful happy heterotopia) (2021, 86). In short, it is as though the fall from the garden is already incorporated in the design of the Congrégation—it was, in other words, bound to happen. For indeed, the "natural" world that Pacôme seeks to recover and be a part of has always already fallen prey to colonial expropriation and exploitation of both women and the land. Her proposal of recovery in the present therefore lies in the idea of a corrected past—a caring agenda that, ironically, leads to the silencing of both the living environment and the women of the Congrégation.

Of course, there is a pre-existing caution expressed in Glissant's understanding of the Return as he addresses with skepticism the idea of recovering a lost past. In *Le discours antillais*, he links "l'obsession de l'Un" (the obsession with the One) with the idea of a return to a singular, exclusionary origin—as such, Glissant explains, "Revenir, c'est consacrer la permanence, la non-relation" (Returning is the acceptance of permanence, of non-relation) ([1981] 1997, 44).[7] This is justified when one considers the fragmented and widely dispersed cultures constitutive of Caribbean history. Looking at the establishment of the Congrégation, there is, for that matter, perhaps already something of a warning in a community confined within an original time-space enclosure, resulting from tracking down all of Charles Débaury's sexual infidelities. A primary condition for the existence of the Congrégation, thus, depends on rehabilitating a foundational family tree that begins with an unfaithful and debauched man (the terms used to refer to Charles Débaury's abuses include "son existence de chien," dog's existence; or "sa vie de débauche," life of debauchery; *MC*, 16–17). Only then will Mère Pacôme be able to "démarrer sa mission" (start her mission) (*MC*, 21)—that is, to organize the confined space of the Congrégation and await the birth of a baby boy in order for the Daughters of Cham to initiate their descent, a somewhat nonevolving, limiting, and heterocentric (in reference to d'Orlando and Harpin's analysis of the novel) prospect, to say the least.

In light of such constricted premises, the silencing of both the living landscape and the women subsequently becomes a condition for the Congrégation to live on, while making all the more apparent Mère Pacôme's recipe for disaster. First, as regards the Daughters of Cham's greenworld: Morne Câpresse fails to perform the promise of *marronnage* (marooning), in the sense of, after Glissant, an escape, a flight from a constrained world toward the possibility of an alternative. In the act of running away, embedded in resistance of the enslaved, marronnage constitutes a strategy of resistance, a deviation from a linear and single historical trajectory. In keeping with the promise of shape-shifting realities linked to past practices of marronnage, Françoise Vergès reclaims the term in the present to refer to "toutes les initiatives, toutes les actions, tous les gestes, les chants, les rituels qui la nuit ou le jour, cachés ou visibles, représentent une promesse radicale" (all the initiatives, actions, gestures, songs, rituals that day and night, hidden or visible, represent a radical promise) (2019b, 37). In this sense, marronnage is closely intertwined with a present that must be questioned and a future that must be imagined. Such practice, following Vergès's definition, does not lose touch with the challenges of the present moment, nor the concrete conceptualization of alternative, livable futures. After Vergès's definition, *marronnage*, thus, not so much operates outside the world (or "hors-monde" to use Ferdinand's expression) but rather continuously interrogates the sustainability of the present for a better, more caring future to be realized. As Marronnes of days past would take flight and become fugitives to resist enslavement under restrictive laws, the act of taking flight in the present may reveal itself both disruptive and creative. Unlike Ferdinand's understanding of marronnage as a "fuite hors-monde" (flight outside the world), the "fugitivity" of yesterday and of today can very much take shape in the belief that the present must be confronted for the future to be different.[8]

But in the case of Pacôme and the Daughters of Cham's escape to the morne, as a consequence of the Congrégation's time-space enclosure, their refusal and exit from what is identified as "le monde d'en bas" or "the world below" is emptied out of its potential for change, for an alternative world. The plantation, although reclaimed from a former béké *planteur* (plantation owner), reproduces the same spatial and temporal restrictions as the colonial plantation. As Glissant explains in *Poétique de la relation*, the plantation as part of the colonial system involves,

> Une organisation socialement pyramidale, confinée dans un lieu clos, fonctionnant apparemment en autarcie mais réellement en dépendance, et dont le mode technique de production est non évolutif parce qu'il est basé sur une structure esclavagiste. (1990, 78)

> An organization formed in a social pyramid, confined within an enclosure, functioning apparently as an autarky but actually dependent, and with a technical mode of production that cannot evolve because it is based on a slave structure. (1997, 63)

Similarly, when Line receives the Congrégation's welcome booklet, she reads,

> En page 2 du livret se déployait un organigramme détaillé. Le graphique représentait la structure pyramidale de la Congrégation. En son sommet, il y avait un portrait de Sainte Mère Pacôme. . . . Dans les pages suivantes, on découvrait une journée type des Filles de Cham ponctuée de prière obligatoires et autres salutations au Soleil. (*MC*, 152–153)
>
> On page 2 of the booklet there was a detailed organization chart representing the pyramidal structure of the Congrégation. At the top there was a portrait of Sainte Mère Pacôme. . . . In the following pages, the Daughters of Cham's typical day was described including frequent mandatory prayers and other greetings to the Sun.

What is Morne Câpresse, then, if not an aspiring autarky presided over by self-anointed Sainte Mère Pacôme and her tightly administered women's garden? In fact, Mère Pacôme's fixation with preplantation (prelapsarian?) natural abundance is what shapes the Congrégation into a strict hierarchical structure, forced to religiously observe its own time-space continuum in order to remain viable.

As the narrator reminds us, the world from which the women of the Congrégation have departed bears the scars of pervasive violence against women—they serve as living testimony to this harsh reality. Moreover, in the world they have left behind, the land too bears the marks of degradation, disfigured by monoculture plantations and contaminated by the continuous use of pesticides and chemical fertilizers (*MC*, 58). The magnitude of exploitation is such that Mère Pacôme appears to have coped with it by seeking refuge, by constructing a sanctuary for both the land and the women. And thus, the Daughters of Cham might have become Marronnes in their present time, yet their marronnage is limited to the initial flight, restrained by the rigid boundaries of a re-created outside-the-world garden—an ideal seemingly unattainable within the polluted world below. Their version of marronnage is, in a way, closer to Ferdinand's understanding of the "fuite Marronne" (Maroon flight) as the impossibility of the garden in the world below is left unconfronted and instead causes removal and enclosure.[9] Furthermore, their transition into the world below, contingent upon the birth of a male child depicted by Pacôme as the next messiah, remains indefinitely postponed. This is due to Pacôme's half-sister, Soeur Lucia, who oversees the "Service de la Santé" (health department), ensuring that no male infants are ever born in the Congrégation by resolutely and secretly committing infanticide on each male newborn. This additional insight into the Congrégation's leadership could serve as yet another ominous sign that the anticipated rescue mission has gone wrong, revealing that the women's community bears ill fruit.

From outside the Congrégation, Morne Câpresse already appears to people as a confined, contained, and possibly perilous place. When Line gets off the bus at the stop "Morne Câpresse," someone comments in passing, "Paraît qu'on n'en revient pas" (I've heard no one comes back from there). Another bystander adds, "On raconte qu'elles sont tenues pis que des esclaves" (I've heard that they are held in captivity worse than slaves) (*MC*, 32). When Line enters the Congrégation, she constitutes an outsider perspective whose narrative voice not only reveals the structuring ploy but also points to the cracks of a failing attempt at healing both women and a ravaged living environment. Line's initiation into the Congrégation, even if motivated by the search for her missing sister, compels the Daughters of Cham to uncover the inner workings of their organization, beginning with the formal protocol that the women observe unchangeably. "C'est le protocole" (We follow protocol). These are the three words that the women of the Congrégation constantly repeat to Line as she is being ordered around. For example, when Line arrives at the morne and tries to show a group of women a photograph of her sister, they interrupt her by explaining that she must discuss this matter with Soeur Lucia first—in other words, she must respect the hierarchy. Meanwhile, the disciplined Daughters of Cham are reciting the same undisturbed welcome: "Bienvenue à la Congrégation des Filles de Cham!" (Welcome to the Daughters of Cham's Congregation!) (*MC*, 73) they say mechanically as Line traverses the morne.

Conversely, everything the reader encounters from Line's internal thoughts or spoken words is completely unfettered in the text, standing in sharp contrast to the silence imposed on the Daughters of Cham. Through Line's unrestrained voice, it becomes possible to interrogate the terms for the recovery of both women and the land as intended by the Congrégation. As Ziethen has analyzed, Line is the Other; as she comes from the world below, she "met en question les pratiques et les idées de Mère Pacôme" (calls into question Mère Pacôme's practices and ideas) and "déclenche [la] chute du système" (causes the demise of the system) (65). To this I would add that disruption comes largely with the deployment of voice, particularly with the retrieval and liberation of voices so far ignored while also questioning the caring foundations of the Congrégation.

If we consider care through the lens of American psychologist Carol Gilligan, who emphasizes attending to voices, particularly those of the most marginalized and invisibilized in society, such attention is demonstrated through Line's expression of self and the voices she makes heard—voices that were, voluntarily or not, censored under Pacôme's rule. In the essay translated in French, "Une voix différente: Un regard prospectif à partir du passé," Gilligan reaffirms that the ethics of care are grounded in voice, in the importance of having a voice, in being listened to with attention and heard. As she has written, "La voix différente est une voix de résistance [aux] dualités et hiérarchies, et l'éthique du care, avec son attention à la voix . . . est l'éthique d'une société démocratique" (The different voice is a voice of resistance against dualities and hierarchies, and the ethics of care, by paying particular attention to voice . . . is the ethics of a democratic society) (2010, 20).[10] In a way, Line's presence among the community of women constitutes resistance as she embodies the abundance of an alternative, a different voice against the limits of a scripted as well as faltering speech.

First, as regards Line's presence, the character provides insight into the stammering of a possibly psychotic matriarch; at an address to the Congrégation, Mère Pacôme announces hesitantly, "Oui, nous ne polluons pas la terre! Nous ensemencons la terre de . . . Vous . . . Chlordécone et les amis de . . . Les maudits sont . . . Pesticides . . . Les anges" (Yes, we do not pollute the Earth! We sow the seeds of . . . You . . . Chlordecone and the friends of . . . The cursed ones are . . . Pesticides . . . Angels) (*MC*, 108). In exposing such incoherent rambling, Line's narrative perspective might already destabilize the ascendancy of Pacôme's voice. Moreover, whether in the form of internal monologue or during conversations with the Daughters of Cham, Line's voice is useful for discerning the workings of a community that reveals itself to be oppressive to women after they have escaped their original plight. For example, as Line is shown around by Soeur Régina, who is in charge of the Service de l'Accueil (the Reception Service), Line delivers an abrasive portrait of the Congrégation:

> "Depuis son arrivée à la Congrégation, elle n'avait fait qu'obéir aux ordres, se plier à la rigidité du fameux protocole. . . . Il n'était plus nécessaire de penser. On pensait à votre place. . . . Tout était programmé. Vous n'aviez plus à vous faire de soucis. Seulement vous soumettre. (*MC*, 95)

> Since she arrived to the Congrégation, she has been following orders, giving in to the rigidity of the notorious protocol. . . . There was no need to think anymore. . . . Someone was doing the thinking for you. . . . Everything was planned. You didn't have to worry anymore. Just to comply.

The world of the Daughters of Cham is here scrutinized from a distant, almost from-above perspective, which allows for the critical interrogations of what has otherwise been normalized. The totalitarian violence and its particular oppressive effect on the voices of the Congrégation's women thus emerges as Line explores what has, in turn, become the "world below."

Line's voice eventually allows for the release of voices that had been previously constrained by Mère Pacôme's monovocal ideology. In terms of what happens at the level of text, placing Line's voice alongside that of Mère Pacôme and her followers creates an alternative narrative avenue, one that makes women's voices resound in all their complexity and diversity. In other words, by being in that space, Line makes known what was already there, shedding light on the parallel lives of the women of the Congrégation. The reader learns, for instance, that Jada ("la grande communicante de la Congrégation") and Divine ("la prêtresse du Service religieux"; *MC*, 194) have started their own businesses in the world below: Jada owns a building in Pointe-à-Pitre and rents out apartments, and Divine runs a few stores that specialize in creole crafts and organic food products (*MC*, 226). As they are being released, the women's voices expose that the descent, at least partially, into the world below has already been initiated—a few women of the Congrégation, who have started to question the viability of Pacôme's project, have, like Jada and Divine, created opportunities for exit, even if not fully, or they have taken control over the fate of the community (for example, Lucia, who refuses the descent from the morne, has ensured its longevity by eliminating every male child).

In a related vein, German economist Albert Hirschman uses the concepts of exit and voice to determine the decline of firms, organizations, and states. Although his exit-voice model originally applied only to the economy, it remains pertinent for acknowledging a dysfunctional system in a noneconomic sense as well. In *Exit, Voice, and Loyalty* (1970), Hirschman identifies exit as the "'direct' way of expressing one's unfavorable view of an organization" (17) and "voice" as "the only way in which dissatisfied customers or members can react whenever the exit option is unavailable" (44). From within the Congrégation, when voice is unavailable to the censored Daughters of Cham, exit prevails, however limited it may be. But through Line's presence in the community voices that might have otherwise remained unknown are granted space within the narrative—which not only unsettles the stability of the Congrégation but also debunks its attempt at giving care to both a damaged living environment and the "filles perdues" outside the world below. Eventually, Mère Pacôme, guided by voices ("les voix des démons," demons' voices, covering "les voix des anges," angels' voices; *MC*, 283) that are not her own, sets her house on fire during a hallucination; the fire then spreads, devastating the garden that had long sustained the community and forcing the Daughters of Cham to retreat back down to "le monde d'en bas" (the world below). Thus, as this discussion has shown, the caring act that Pacôme sets out to perform is unsuccessful because it results in silencing the land she intends to reclaim and replenish as well as the women she means to heal. As Régina laconically observes, "Le ver était déjà dans le fruit" (the worm was already in the fruit) (*MC*, 162). The land that the Daughters of Cham seek to recover has been forever damaged, and the women that Pacôme is resolved to heal have been profoundly marked by violence, starting with Pacôme herself, described from the start of the novel as "une négresse brisée, là-bas en France, enfermée dans un bocal sous terre" (a broken Negress, over there in France, locked in a booth in an underground train station) (*MC*, 24).

This failed act of care also shows that the history of colonial violence in the region and the legacy of exploitation of both the land and human lives (especially women in the novel) must not be ignored or dismissed. Rather, the wounded human voices must resound, the past and present violent realities of the territories they inhabit must be known, and the challenges they present must be collectively acknowledged. Through Mère Pacôme's Congrégation project, we see the struggle of the caregiver to formulate an appropriate act of care to recover from a traumatic past, but there is meaning in the fall. For indeed, can such a catastrophe ("cette catastrophe"; *MC*, 292) act as a template in reverse for caring for the wounded women and land, and more generally for caring relations across human and nonhuman worlds? What if the proposal to heal, to care in the present, was not so much contained in the *re*covered garden of the Daughters of Cham but rather in the irrevocable fall from the garden? The term "catastrophe," used in the text at the moment of the community's fall, quite fittingly comes from the Greek *kata*, which means a movement down or downward. As *Morne Câpresse* concludes, the significance of returning to a world scarred by the legacy of colonial spoliation and devastation remains unclear, as does any potential of returning to Earth that may exist behind or beyond the act of falling. However, as readers, we are perhaps left with an invitation to contemplate the practices of care that can be salvaged in a world that has turned into a "décharge sauvage" (a wild garbage dump) (*MC*, 58).

And what does the world below look like? In the "wild garbage dump" that the Daughters of Cham-to-be wish to escape by joining the Congrégation, the land is described as being ravaged by pesticides, chemical fertilizers, and concrete. In a rambling speech, Mère Pacôme alludes in particular to chlordecone (also known under its brand name Kepone), a toxic pesticide used in banana plantations to eradicate weevils between the years 1972 and 1993 in Guadeloupe and Martinique.

Although chlordecone was banned in the United States after the Kepone environmental scandal in Hopewell, Virginia, in 1975 and was ruled carcinogenic in 1979 by the International Agency for Research on Cancer, the French government only banned its use in 1990—and the remaining stock of the product was still being used in banana plantations in the French Caribbean until 1993.[11] In the graphic narrative *Tropiques toxiques* (2020; hereafter *TT*), Jessica Oublié recounts how she learned of chlordecone poisoning when she moved to Guadeloupe in February 2018 to be closer to the maternal side of her family. After that, Oublié started to investigate the historical, political, and economic circumstances that led to the use of the pesticide as well as the harmful effects of chlordecone exposure to both the human and nonhuman worlds. In short, *Tropiques toxiques* constitutes an intimate dive into people's lived experiences in the French Caribbean, paired with the elaboration of attentive scientific knowledge around the contamination caused by chlordecone and its continued effects—a polyphonic and multiperspectival documentary narrative that the comic form makes possible and visible.

Chlordecone is an extremely toxic, nonbiodegradable substance that affects soil and waterways as well as all forms of life (human and nonhuman) and persists in the environment on average between seventy and 700 years,[12] depending on the type of soil. Oublié's investigative work has highly contributed to the visibility of chlordecone pollution, shedding light on environmentally damaging practices that endanger human and nonhuman health, food, and water sustainability as well as traditional lifestyles such as the Creole garden.

Historically, the Creole garden remains ambivalent because it is rooted in the legacy of colonial oppression. Indeed, aside from plantation monocultures, gardening served as a vital means of subsistence and survival for enslaved individuals, who had to cultivate their own food to sustain themselves.[13] Looking at Glissant's theorization of the *jardin créole* in Manthia Diawara's documentary *Édouard Glissant: One World in Relation* (2010), Jeannine Murray-Román (2022) quotes from Glissant's definition of the jardin créole at length. She reminds us that the latter was originally cultivated by the enslaved after their labors at the margins of the plantation, often clandestinely, to produce a variety of fruit and vegetables and therefore maintain provision grounds. In her study on gardening practices during colonial times, anthropologist Catherine Benoît (2015) also argues that the garden participates in the affirmation of identity as well as the appropriation and formation of territory, revealing life-maintaining relations between people and their environment.[14] Still in conversation with Glissant, Murray-Román presents a similar understanding of the *jardin créole* by identifying it as a "structure for caring more" (2022, 86) as it participates in a "life-sustaining web" (79) and creates "conditions for heterogeneous distribution and mutual protection" (85). The *jardin créole*, as conceptualized by scholars and writers such as

Benoît, Glissant, and Murray-Román, undoubtedly evokes a colonial lineage. However, as this practice has passed down through generations it may also have enabled individuals and local communities to maintain cultivating practices that promote self-sufficiency, greater diversification, and mutual distribution.

And yet, in the contemporary context, as Oublié chronicles the effects of chlordecone contamination on both human and nonhuman lives as well as habitats, the *jardin créole* is represented as polluted, which results, at least at first, in more impossibility than possibility. As the *jardin créole* appears visually in multiple instances in the graphic narrative, we see that there is a temporal discontinuity between gardening practices that used to be possible and the impossibility of the garden in the present, combined with the degradation of human health. Given this temporal rupture, the graphic narrative develops a color code to distinguish different time periods, especially as regards the disruption of cultural practices such as gardening.

Showing the relationship between exposure to chlordecone and the risk of prostate cancer, Oublié introduces Monsieur Louison who was diagnosed with prostate cancer (Figure 6). In one panel, Louison appears in the doctor's office on the day his cancer is diagnosed; as he moves to the window of the office and reminisces, the reader travels through space to see him in the next panel looking at his home garden (*TT*, 106–107). In the left-hand side of the top panel, Monsieur Louison is drawn with vivid colors and says, "J'ador*ais* jardiner, j'utilis*ais* plein de produits, des désherbants, des fongicides, le tout sans protection" (I love*d* gardening, I *would* use a lot of products, weedkillers and fungicide, all of this without protection) (emphasis mine) as he observes a past version of himself, drawn with more faded colors, tending the garden with his bare hands (*TT*, 107). The juxtaposition of the past and the present not only makes clear visually the causal relationship between chlordecone exposure and the man's cancer diagnosis but also points to a gardening practice that cannot continue in the present as a result of the long-term pollution of the French Antilles.

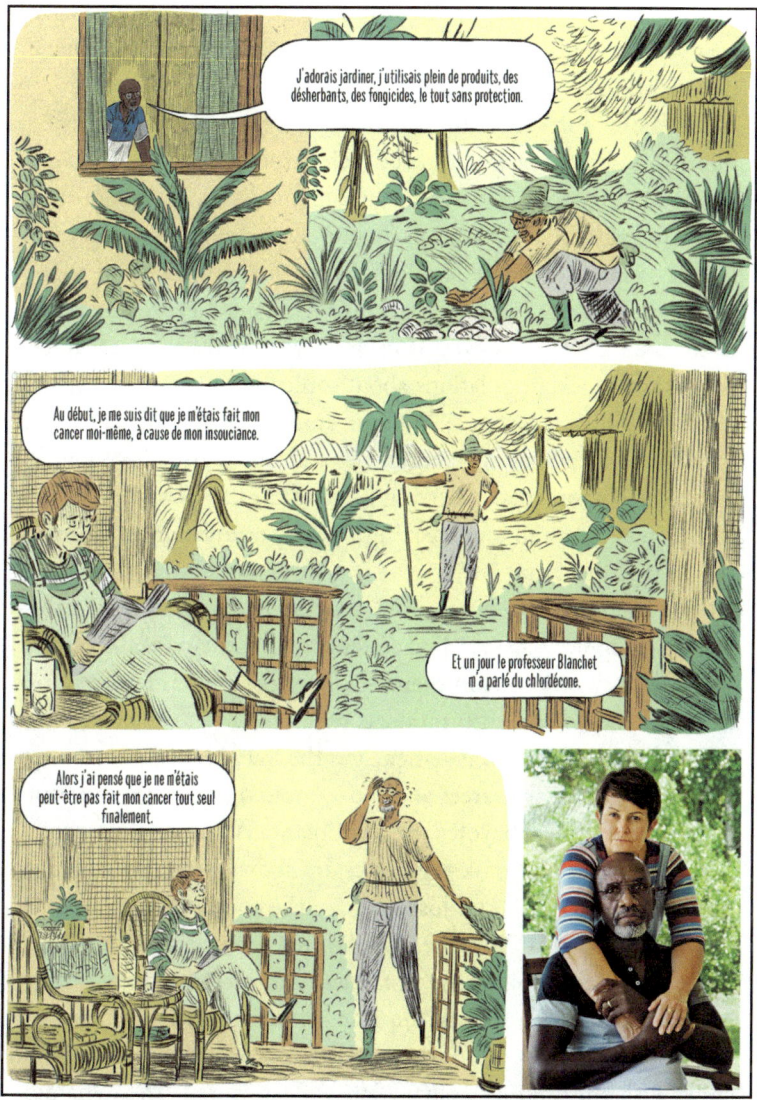

FIG. 6. *Tropiques toxiques*, page 107 © Steinkis / Les Escales, 2020

Text from left to right, in order in which the speech bubbles appear: "I used to love gardening, I used a lot of products, herbicides, fungicides, all without protection." "At first, I thought I had caused my own cancer, because of my carelessness." "And one day, Professor Blanchet talked to me about chlordecone." "So I thought that maybe I hadn't caused my cancer all by myself after all."

The *jardin créole* also undoubtedly integrates a rich biodiversity that reflects both a form of craft as well as long-lasting culinary traditions—both are being forcibly discontinued because of chlordecone poisoning. In the present of the graphic narrative, interruption if not termination of such gardening practices is similarly visually signaled, suggesting that remodeling cultivation and culinary traditions is required. Oublié recounts her meeting with a local couple, Ghislaine and José, living on the grounds of a former banana plantation (Figure 7). She had joined Fred, a member of the program Jardins Familiaux (Jafa), who works to raise awareness among local populations about soil contamination by chlordecone.[15] During his visit, Fred informs the couple that the soil where they grow their own vegetables and fruit is heavily contaminated with chlordecone, alerting them to the dangers of exposure to the pesticide and emphasizing the importance of rethinking their gardening habits.

The interaction between Fred and the landowners, especially José, is fraught, at least at first: after showing them results of the analysis of chlordecone in their soil, Fred lists the different crops that they should no longer produce, especially root vegetables such as ginger, sweet potato, malanga, and the like. He tells them they should refocus on fruit trees and above-ground vegetables and fruit such as pineapple, chayote, and chili plant. While Fred is speaking, the several high-risk vegetables are shown being crossed out on the page (*TT*, 91), and José's face in the corner shows increasing disbelief and annoyance. While Fred emphasizes the indispensable, vital role of the *jardin créole* in fostering healthy eating habits, he also highlights the impact of enduring legacies of harm on the lived environment, thereby complicating relationships with the land and particularly affecting the "the dynamic practices of care," as Murray-Román puts it (2022, 82), that may emerge from gardening.

The fact remains that people like José and Ghislaine express a desire for rootedness to the land they inhabit—the section of the documentary graphic narrative dedicated to their story concludes

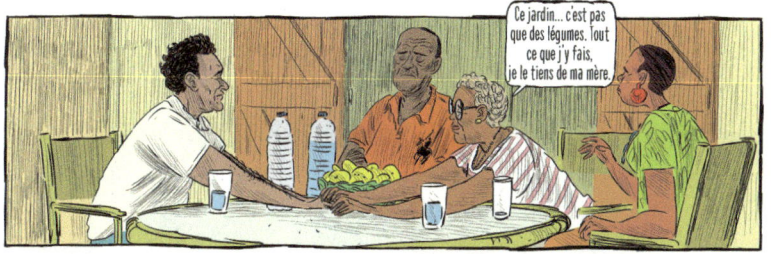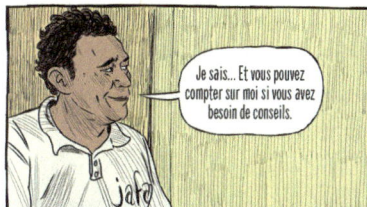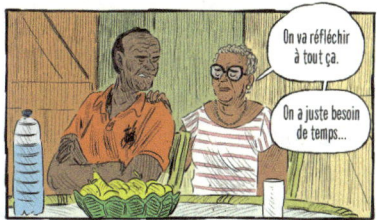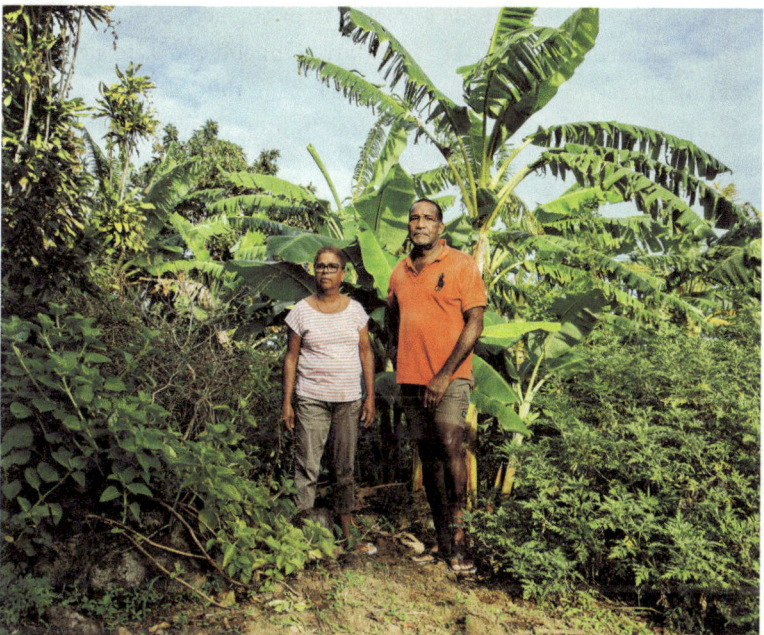

FIG. 7. *Tropiques toxiques*, page 93 © Steinkis / Les Escales, 2020

Text from left to right, in order in which the speech bubbles appear: "This garden is not just about vegetables. Everything I do here, I learned from my mother." "I know . . . And you can count on me if you need advice." "We'll think about all of this." "We just need time."

with a photograph where they appear grounded in the landscape as they are surrounded with the dense vegetation of their homegrown garden, their feet barely apparent. Yet the question now arises of how to care for themselves as well as their land, for the knowledge of contaminated soil gets in the way of their inhabitation of the land and can hardly be ignored.

The photographic conclusion to the segment concerning José and Ghislaine also conveys the resolute commitment of local populations to remain grounded in the land they inhabit while concurrently thinking about ways to sustain life, their own as well as the nonhuman life forms surrounding them. "On va réfléchir à tout ça. On a juste besoin de temps" (We're going to think about all this. We just need time) Ghislaine tells Fred after he has presented them with ways to cultivate and raise their chickens differently in contaminated areas (*TT*, 93). In a way, to inhabit comes to signify caring from within one's dwelling place, as in the case of José and Ghislaine for whom to inhabit means finding (new) ways for life to go on in the land they inhabit.

When we look at the etymology of the verb "to inhabit," it becomes clear that the self may ideally be thought of in relation to the place where one resides, momentarily or for a prolonged period. "To inhabit," from the Latin *inhabitare*, means "to dwell in," which itself relates to the idea of making a home, having residence in a place.[16] Yet in an environment contaminated by chlordecone (or any other pollutant for that matter), the possibility of inhabiting, of creating an idea of home, somewhere to belong, is founded on a compromised reality.[17] For a long-standing practice such as the *jardin créole* to subsist, caring is not only located in the persistence of inhabitation but also in tuning in to voices and practices that are working to re-create an idea of home in a damaged world.

During the first meeting between Oublié and Luc Multigner, the epidemiologist observes "On ne peut pas évacuer les gens et leur proposer de tout recommencer ailleurs" (We cannot evacuate everyone and suggest that they start over elsewhere), and he concludes with a question: "Comment apprendre à vivre avec un problème majeur de pollution environnementale?" (How do we learn to live with a major issue of environmental pollution?) (*TT*, 38). *Tropiques toxiques* only integrates voices and bodies grounded in the land they inhabit—it is never a question of whether to leave or not. Rather the graphic narrative foregrounds local and individual attempts to redress government inaction or irresolute attitude as regards chlordecone contamination.[18] Especially in the last two chapters of the graphic narrative ("En attendant, kisa *nou* fè?" (Meanwhile, what can *we* do?) (emphasis mine), and "Repenser les ponts possibles entre tous les êtres vivants et édifier le monde d'après" (Rethinking the possible bridges between living beings and building the world of tomorrow), *grounded*ness in the land (in the sense of being a part of it) is achieved through the interaction of image and text with photography. These photos are most often interspersed with drawn images, and speech bubbles are adjacent to individuals. In a way, these are individuals who are momentarily extracted from their present realities to inhabit the page and speak for themselves.

For readers, these individuals transform from characters drawn on a page into fully realized, living people. In an interview with the *Kwazman Vwa* collective in March 2021, Oublié noted that, although she made sure to remind people that *Tropiques toxiques* is a documentary graphic narrative based on "real-life" testimonies, she received feedback on social media from readers who believed it was a work of fiction.[19] The integration of photographic individuals in the graphic narrative is important to concretize their relationship to the land, one that is deploying caring practices toward others, the self, and the land, one that demonstrates awareness that the *reality* of chlordecone contamination is endangering the continuation of life as it has been lived.

As Glissant observes, the relationship with the land is threatened, but in light of what is captured by the photographic image, alongside testimonial evidence from people directly impacted by chlordecone poisoning, the situation is not one of alienation from the land.[20] Instead, photography is mobilized to affirm these individuals' presence in the land and their renewed desire, as well as struggle, to inhabit it, to "render them fleshly individuals with presence and affect" (Campt 2017, 91). Again, there is great potential in the idea of inhabiting when it is reconciled with the prospect of living with care after or in light of the damage, of inventing or reinventing new ways of inhabitation in a polluted land. Here I take the liberty of adapting Tanella Boni's interpretation of the French verb *habiter*, as the act of "inventer de la vie là où il n'y en a pas" (inventing life where there is none) (2018, 9). Framed in this manner, "habiter" revitalizes the prospect of establishing a sense of home, reinstating the term's association with its etymological roots. Illustrating the possibility to develop a sense of place despite chlordecone poisoning, the photographed individuals in the graphic narrative include local farmers such as Michel in Baillif, Guadeloupe, or Alex Toly in Trois-Rivières, who have reimagined their farming practices to circumvent environmental contamination (*TT*, 204). Toly explains, for example, that he is now raising chickens above ground to secure eggs without chlordecone—one way of caring for his own health as well as that of others.

The reader also finds photographs that capture moments of collective gathering, where individuals voice their concerns and frustrations about chlordecone poisoning and urgently seek solutions in the present to ensure a sustainable future. We see, for example, a few members of the collective Lyannaj pou dépolyé Matinik gathered during one of their weekly meetings at the Maison des Syndicats de Fort-de-France; they discuss consumer trust, state financial aid to farmers, and consumption of local foods (*TT*, 205).[21] Another series of photographs shows a gathering organized by the bookstore Kazabul at Garage Popular in Fort-de-France on the theme "Quand BD et société se rencontrent: chronique d'un quotidien d'un genre nouveau" (When comics and society meet: chronicling the new everyday) (*TT*, 214), which Oublié moderated. The attendees were invited to open up about how their lives have been impacted by chlordecone poisoning. The purpose of this meeting was not so much to think (yet) about alternative lifestyles in a newfound polluted reality but rather to create a space where individuals may become visible and heard—a space that is consolidated in the graphic narrative through the means of photography. The photographic image, juxtaposed with drawn images, thus both evidences the prospect of groundedness in the land, of a life-sustaining way of inhabitation, and also shows individuals who by taking ownership of their voice and image compel us to reckon with the devastating impact of long-standing neglect.

Because, in fact, what is chlordecone pollution in the French Antilles if not the blatant consequence of uncaring practices toward the lives and the living environment of those perceived as distant, as Other? In an interview on the theme of "Antilles empoisonnées: Le scandale du chlordécone," as part of the podcast series "Kiffe ta race" hosted by Rokhaya Diallo and Grace Ly (2020), Oublié suggested that, from the perspective of hexagonal France, the overseas territories remain comfortably distanced and are perceived as socioculturally "other." Oublié's verbalization of such perception includes expressions such as "on ferme les yeux" (we pretend not to notice) or "c'est loin là-bas, qu'ils se débrouillent entre eux" (it's far out there, have them deal with their problems themselves). For in that case, to care for the lives of others and the living environment appears insignificant compared with a renewed concern for the steady export of Antillean bananas and the profitability associated with it, especially for békés who, to this day, control a large part of import-export as well as agricultural lands in the French Caribbean.[22]

There is a lack of care, or what Joan Tronto designates as a "caring deficit," in overlooking the human and environmental cost of the profitability of the few.[23] There is a lack of care in what has so far gone unspoken or unrecognized, in what has been deceivingly toned down. The graphic narrative helps to locate this lack of care in the persistent dismissal of the toxicity of chlordecone on the part, largely, of government officials. We see in one panel a few of the key players who over several decades authorized the extended use of chlordecone despite its known adverse effects (*TT*, 143): Jacques Chirac (Minister of Agriculture and Rural Development, 1972–1973), Édith Cresson (Minister of Agriculture, 1981–1983), and Henri Nallet (Minister of Agriculture, 1988–1990) are depicted covering, respectively, their eyes, their ears, or their mouth in clear denial. To use such iconography is deeply ironic: the reference to the three wise monkeys who see no evil, hear no evil, speak no evil is applied to those who have turned a blind eye to knowledge about the chlordecone causing catastrophic and lasting damage to the environment as well as the human and nonhuman lives that inhabit it.

Throughout the graphic narrative, the visual presence and voices of those who have for a long time afforded not to care is interspersed with those grounded in the world below (if they have not escaped like the Daughters of Cham), leaving an impression of proximity and potentially creating the conditions within which one—including the reader—could see and hear the other. Such assemblage of individual voices and bodies aspires to trade distance for proximity, uncaring for attentiveness. In the end, what potential, we must ask, lies in the act of reflecting collectively on how to care adequately and expansively in a wounded world?

Imagining an exchange in a reconstituted civil society at the end of the graphic narrative, Oublié already dares to create a collective space where the overlooked reality of chlordecone contamination is recognized and where thus far dismissed voices may be heard (Figure 8). All may then come together to untangle the historical legacy of uncaring toward human and nonhuman lives as well as their living environment, which has been perceived as distant. All may come to reflect on the adequacy or inadequacy of practices of care in the present for a life-sustaining future to be realized. Among the large assembly gathered to interrogate our ways of inhabiting the world, we see and listen to scholars and writers Dominique Bourg, Malcolm Ferdinand, Cynthia Fleury, and Tanella Boni seated in the first row (*TT*, 221–225). Here, even

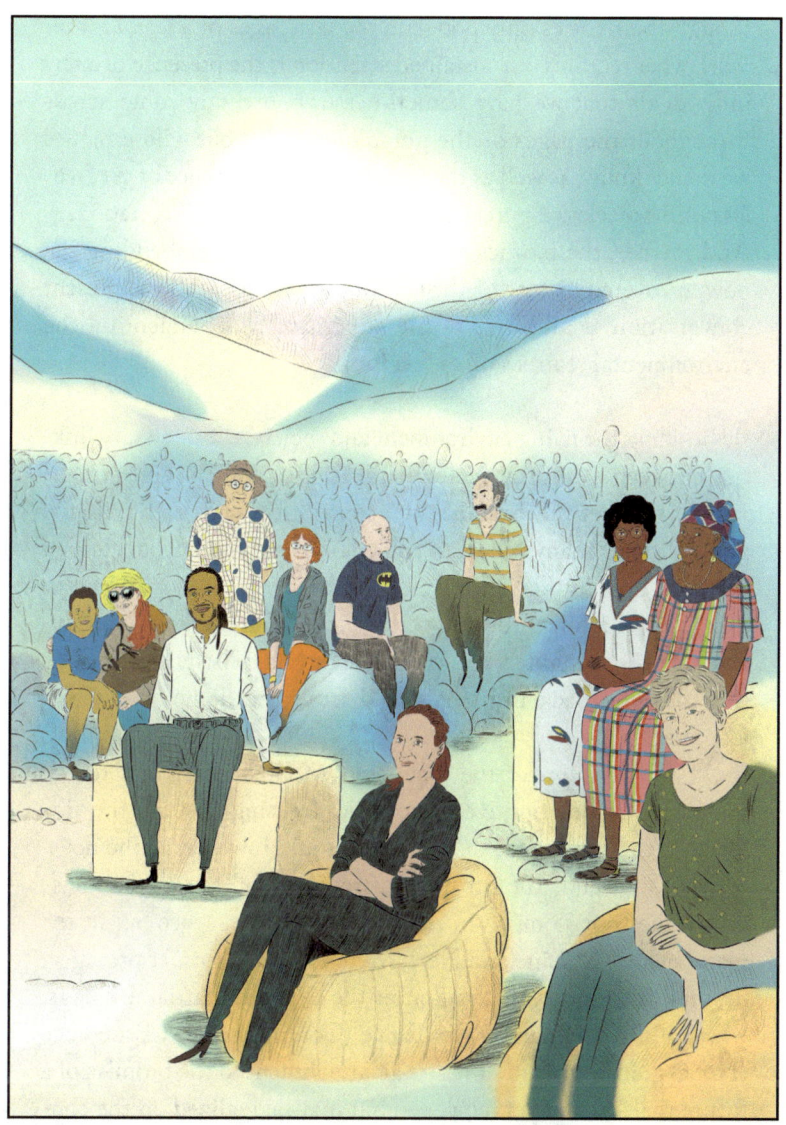

FIG. 8. *Tropiques toxiques*, page 221 © Steinkis / Les Escales, 2020

though their voices only populate the last pages of *Tropiques toxiques*, what requires our sustained attention is the presence of a few individuals that we have sometimes unknowingly come across throughout the pages of the graphic narrative but whose names we do not know, as well as the even more faint presence of yet faceless and voiceless figures lined up behind them (*TT*, 220–221). And further, the mornes surround the assembly, embedding the now uncovered history of the Caribbean landscape in the present conversation as all forms of life are critically dependent on the environmental realities of the region.

By bridging the living environment and society, the necessary linkage between a healthy ecology and healthy human and nonhuman lives effectively becomes apparent. In the end, sketching the possibility for many others to come join this assembly, to claim a body left unidentified and a voice left unheard, extends an invitation to inhabit forcefully the world below. Would it be so conceivable that the Daughters of Cham come to claim body and voice as they descend back into the world from the flames of Morne Câpresse?

In *Morne Câpresse*, the Daughters of Cham first find refuge in Mère Pacôme's fugitive greenworld, refusing to suffer the violence of their existence in a ravaged land. However, as the novel comes to an end, the prospect of recovery of the land, if sustained, lies not so much in the enclosed garden space but in the world below. As Line and Neel, Mère Pacôme's former protégée, descend the morne, they call after the deposed matriarch's dogs, who are fittingly named Confiance (Confidence) and Espérance (Hope) going outward. There is an attachment to the promise of a future that has not yet happened but may be realized on the condition that these two women replant themselves in the environment once dismissed by the Daughters of Cham. "Il fallait juste s'accrocher à cette espérance, avoir confiance" (They had to hold on to this hope, have confidence) (*MC*, 324)—the novel concludes with these words. Line and Neel's disposition is one that shows their commitment to the attentive labor of creating an alternative reality, one that reflects their active and individual role in ensuring that care is restored. Their resounding voices may eventually populate the assembly formed by a civil society invested in the labor of caring, as it is portrayed in *Tropiques toxiques*.

4
Rebellious Care, or Deconstructing the Myth of the *Poto-mitan* Woman

"Fem-n cé chataign, m'hom-n cé fouyapin" (Woman is a chestnut, Man is a breadfruit). The Kreyòl proverb, quoted in Maryse Condé's *La parole des femmes* (1979), is evocative of the strength and resilience historically attributed to Caribbean women during and since slavery. In the context of slavery, the 1685 *Code Noir*, specifically law XIII, establishes the woman–child pair in bondage, stripping enslaved men of rights to their offspring and imposing onto enslaved women the task of reproductive labor.[1] This historical burden has been interpreted over time as the fact of Caribbean women's tenacity and strength in adversity, reframing gendered oppression as a testimony to women's resilience. Hence, proverbs like "Fem-n cé chataign, m'hom-n cé fouyapin" serve as manifestation and consolidation of this enduring legacy of slavery. Condé explains the meaning of the metaphor: the chestnut when it falls to the ground "délivre un grand nombre de petits fruits à écorce dure" (yields a large number of thick-skinned fruits), unlike the breadfruit which "se répand en une purée blanchâtre que le soleil ne tarde pas à rendre nauséabonde" (spreads into a whitish mush that quickly starts to emit a pungent smell under the sun) (1979, 4). The image of the chestnut provides an apt metaphor for suffering (the fallen fruit) but also regrowth and abundance. Transposed onto women's experience, the reproductive body of the chestnut symbolizes the resilience, strength, and self-sacrifice associated with the woman-mother in Caribbean contexts (4).

The attributes captured in the chestnut archetype are also reflected in the prevailing cultural perception of women as *poto-mitan* in Caribbean societies. Etymologically, the term "poto-mitan" is a compound word formed by *poto* "pillar" and *mitan* "middle," and it means "the very strength"; the term "poto-mitan" refers literally to the round central pillar that supports the frame of a Vodou temple.[2] Metaphorically, the image of the *poto-mitan*, existing alongside expressions such as *femme matador* (the fighting woman) or *fanm doubout* (standing woman), expresses women's centrality in society and, more particularly, the essential role they play within the family structure. However, this image also produces constricting conditions under which women must organize their social, domestic, and more largely feminine existence. In Nadine Lefaucheur's sociological study, "Situations monoparentales à la Martinique et idéal sacrificiel du potomitan," the single mothers she interviewed view the sociocultural expectation to uphold the family as "un piège pour les femmes" (a trap for women), describing it as involving "trop de responsabilités" (too many responsibilities) and being "très, trop dur à supporter au quotidien" (very, too hard to bear on a daily basis) (34). When integrated to a matrifocal relational system, women and girls inherit a glorified imaginary of resilience, self-sacrifice, and devotion from the female figures who came before them.[3] Clearly, this ideal is being called into question, making the *poto-mitan* the caring figure par excellence to challenge.

In this chapter, I thus start by exploring a refusal of the relegation to care as defined by the *poto-mitan* archetype, introducing the concept of rebellious care through my analysis of Fabienne Kanor's novel *D'eaux douces* (Fresh waters, 2004; hereafter *DD*). In Kanor's novel, the main protagonist, Frida, interrogates a cycle of self-resignation that she inherited from her mother, who encouraged her from childhood to be self-reliant, self-effacing, and nurturing in relation to men. Eventually Frida violently breaks the cycle by murdering her lover, Eric, and killing herself. In analyzing Frida's actions in the light of rebellious care, this chapter argues that *D'eaux douces* shows both the limits of a destructive cycle passed on through generations of women as well as the necessity to imagine a path away from the constraints of a pressing responsibility to care after the *poto-mitan* for women.

I then juxtapose this example of rebellious care with Gaël Octavia's novel *La bonne histoire de Madeleine Démétrius* (Madeleine Démétrius's good story, 2020; hereafter *BH*) in order to examine emancipation from the figure of the *poto-mitan* to a reclamation of vulnerability and empathy. Indeed, Octavia's novel opens with an encounter between the narrator-protagonist, a writer who left Martinique to settle in hexagonal France, and her long-lost high school friend, Madeleine Démétrius. Démétrius entrusts her friend with a troubling story from her childhood. Through a dive into the past, the narrative peels away the layers of fictionalization of the woman pillar across generations to expose the concept's fallacy as well as lay bare its profound impact on the distribution of caregiving responsibilities. Considering these two novels conjointly, I argue that while Kanor's novel shows the bankruptcy of the *poto-mitan* cultural model, Octavia's novel supports competing representations of women in their relations to each other, to male figures, and to those who come after them.

Kanor opens her novel with the conclusion of the story—Frida announces the murder of Eric and her imminent suicide matter-of-factly: "Je m'appelle Frida, je viens de tuer un homme et je m'apprête à me faire sauter la cervelle" (My name is Frida, I just killed a man and I'm about to shoot myself in the head) (*DD*, 7). Kanor also does not seek to dissimulate the interpretation of her protagonist's actions; in an interview with scholar Gladys M. Francis, she states, "La fin [de *D'eaux douces*] est heureuse. Il ne s'agit pas d'une mort, mais d'une renaissance" (The novel has a happy ending. It is not a story about death, but about rebirth) (2016, 284)—a perspective that has since been relayed in the scholarship about Kanor's text (Francis 2017; Vété-Congolo 2015). There has, in fact, been a great deal of critical interest in this particular novel (including Larose 2007; Persson 2017, and Sadai 2009, in addition to the scholars previously mentioned). Building on the work of these scholars, I add that *D'eaux douces* is a work that substantiates the connection between care and oppression. As I will show, Kanor's narrative reveals the forms of oppression that the matrilineal legacy of the *poto-mitan* supports, impacting not only Frida but also Eric and leading up to the protagonist's suffocation and eventual radically subversive act.

Early on in *D'eaux douces*, Frida grapples with her mother's teachings which pervade the text, instructing the protagonist on "good" conduct. Her mother's voice is one that admonishes through free indirect speech, advocating Frida's self-effacement. "Maman dit qu'il ne faut jamais déballer ce que l'on a sur le coeur. . . . Bien se frotter la coucoune à l'eau claire. Ne pas raconter ses affaires. Ne jamais attirer l'attention sur soi" (Mom says to *never* say what's weighing on your heart. To clean your genitals well with clean water. To *never* talk about your problems. To *never* draw attention to yourself) (*DD*, 11–207, emphases mine). In effect, these constraints exemplify the practices of silencing and suppression inherited by women matrilineally. The teachings Frida receives from her mother were passed down through her grandmother—"c'est sa propre mère qui le lui a appris" (it was her own mother who taught her)—to the extent that both maternal figures merge, shaping the path to domestic existence as "une bonne épouse, une bonne mère, une bonne à tout faire" (a good wife, a good mother, a good maid) (*DD*, 12–13). Each qualifying term is intricately connected, culminating in the figure of the maid who constitutes their matrilineal heritage, therefore marking this legacy of caregiving (being a mother and a wife) as oppression.[4]

In her discussion of the Caribbean family, scholar Leighan Renaud (2020) encourages us to look in the direction of the matrifocal family to consider networks of love and support among women, thus avoiding the "model of the nuclear family" and refusing also to focus principally on male figures, whether present, absent, or marginal.[5] But while honoring the networks of love that may emerge from the centrality of women in their roles as mothers, grandmothers, and "othermothers," as Renaud puts it, we need also to think about the underlying forms of psychological coercion and repression that may exist within what could otherwise be idealized as a non-normative, non-nuclear family structure. For indeed, in *D'eaux douces* the specific model of womanhood to which Frida is heiress produces an authoritarian matrifocal community practicing (self-)censorship. In Frida's case, her mother is the executor of a violent and repressive legacy. The character describes in detail the metaphorical actions of the "castrating mother" ("mère castratrice" in the novel; *DD*, 86) as she reflects on her fraught relationship with her romantic partner, Eric, in adulthood: "maman fantôme me tire la langue, me prie d'ouvrir grande la bouche pour me faire avaler son histoire" (my ghost mother pulls out my tongue, asks that I open my mouth wide to make me swallow her history) (*DD*, 25). Frida falls prey to this haunting legacy of women's silent forbearance, resilience, and subjugation as her mother's voice resonates into her adult years, molding the woman she has become. However, the voice is itself not really her mother's but one that generations of women have internalized. As such, whether a conscious "victim" (victim) or not (Persson 2017, 75), Frida's mother repeats a model of predatory motherhood that establishes the habit of suffering and self-effacement.

Indeed, Frida's portrayal of her relationship with her mother from her childhood days introduces an emotionally abusive dynamic, of which the devouring mother becomes the epitome. "Il faut souffrir pour être belle" (One must suffer to be beautiful), Frida's mother tells her daughter as she forcefully combs her hair during childhood (*DD*, 178). The dialogue's structure in this scene replicates that of the scene between the child and the wolf in the grandmother's bed in the children's tale "Little Red Riding Hood." "Maman, que vous avez de longues mains, que vos ongles sont affûtés, que votre voix a changé!" (Mom, what long hands you have, what sharp nails you have, how different your voice sounds!), Frida starts. She continues, "Que vos gestes sont brusques, que votre peigne blesse, que votre sourire est étrange! Silence. Mère va frapper. Maman veut me tuer" (What harsh movements you make, how much your comb hurts, what a strange smile you have! Silence. Mother is going to hit. Mom wants to kill me) (*DD*, 178). The literal and metaphorical retelling of such an archetypal predator–prey relationship highlights the ways in which the individual, be it Frida or her mother, is subsumed within a pervasive and prescriptive cycle of matrilineal repression and violence.

This cycle also has an impact on male children. In *D'eaux douces*, Eric represents the other side of these markedly gendered matrilineal teachings. Even before Frida meets Eric, Afro-Caribbean masculinity is described as inherently damaging, influenced, at least in part, by "un instinct de coq" (a rooster's instinct) and nurtured by overprotective mothers (referred to as "amour de poule" (in the novel, overprotective motherly love; *DD*, 28).[6] The amplification of these hypernormative masculinist tendencies shapes in *D'eaux douces* what Véronique Larose defines as a "homme prédateur, toujours en chasse. Jamais repu" (a predatory man, always on the hunt, never satisfied) (2007, 6.2), linking unrestrained sexuality to the affirmation of masculinity.[7] Influenced by the widespread image of adulterous Afro-Caribbean men, Frida's mother taught her from a young age to be cautious around Black men and to avoid seeing them as potential romantic partners (*DD*, 109). Interestingly, in the interview with scholar Gladys M. Francis, Kanor's reflections on her own upbringing echoed a similar distrust of Black men instilled in her during childhood: "J'ai également grandi dans la peur de l'homme noir. Ma mère nous mettait souvent en garde contre les infidélités et la méchanceté du Noir" (I also grew up in fear of Black men. My mother also warned us to watch out for the infidelities and maliciousness of Black men) (*DD*, 275–276).

Like Kanor's mother, Frida's mother would repeat ad libitum to her "Méfie-toi du nègre" (Beware the Negro), which may seem a justified warning in light of Eric's future infidelities (*DD*, 83). For soon enough Frida learns that Eric is a serial adulterer—the third-person omniscient narrator recounts the character's sexual predation: "Éric a été loup-garou. . . . Il avait mangé-mangé-mangé. . . . De la Guyanaise teint-goyave à l'Asiatique peau douce, il en avait soupé des femmes sans prendre le temps de tout digérer" (Eric has behaved like a werewolf. . . . He has eaten-eaten-eaten. . . . From the glowy-skinned Guianian to the soft-skinned Asian, he had consumed many women without taking the time to digest all of them" (*DD*, 83–84). For Eric, engaging in sexual promiscuity has become the expression of his pursuit of freedom ("Je veux être libre, Frida, me sentir léger comme une plume" (I want to be free, Frida, to feel as light as a feather) (*DD*, 166). However, his perceived "success" in achieving a male-centric form of emancipation ultimately leaves Frida feeling defeated and abandoned: "J'attends ma mort, je l'espère" (I wait for my death, I hope for it), Frida admits (*DD*, 185). Eric has become a life-sucking wolf as well.

Eric's infidelity signifies the demise of Frida's hope of reinventing the Antillean couple with him, her hope of overcoming the historical impossibility of family or relationship formation for descendants of enslaved people. For Frida, the foundation of a new Antillean nation is inextricably tied to what Tina Harpin describes as her "rêverie d'une nouvelle union des couples" (dream of a new union of couples) (2017, 109), highlighting a presumed connection between heterosexual Black romance and the potential for historical redress. Speaking to the history of the heteronormative couple within Caribbean plantation societies, Kathleen Gyssels (2008) justly reminds us that, amid nativist and antifamily politics (one may also think of Glissant's use of the term "antifamille"—antifamily—in *Le discours antillais*, [1981] 1997, 166), "hommes et femmes étaient écartés en tant que couples, en tant que parents responsables de leurs enfants, car la cellule familiale était considérée comme l'éventuelle cause d'insubordination et de révolte" (men and women could not exist as couples, as parents responsible for their children, because the family unit was considered the possible cause of insubordination and revolt) (1.1).

Through her relationship with Eric, Frida sought to disrupt the antifamily relationship model that slavery and colonialism instituted; she refuses to be confined by gender and sexual stereotypes. But instead the revolutionary potential of their love story is undermined when Eric gives in to historically prescribed normative traits. As if reciting from memory, the narrative voice states that Afro-Caribbean manhood means,

> [Être] capable de coquer dix femmes à la minute. De fabriquer des mensonges cent fois plus gros que lui. De voler ta vertu sans prendre de plaisir. . . . Est nègre qui te dit A et pense B. Qui te jure B et pense A. . . . Qui disparaît sans scrupule. Revient sans commentaire. . . . Te fait cinq gosses dans le dos. (*DD*, 79)

> Being capable of sleeping with ten women per minute. Of making up lies a hundred times bigger than himself. Of stealing your virtue without taking pleasure. The Negro says A to you but thinks B. Swears A to you but thinks B. . . . Disappears with no qualms. Comes back without explanation. . . . Has five children behind your back.

This inherited masculinity perverts any other way of being and reverts the couple back to their battle of the sexes—because, after all, "nos hommes ne sont pas fiables. La plupart d'entre eux manquent de principes et de courage" (our men are not reliable. Most of them lack principles and courage) (*DD*, 121). Then what can a woman do except always keep her defenses ready?

In fact, following Eric's infidelity, Marlène, a friend of Frida, introduces her to a self-proclaimed expert in matters of love, the Ministress of Love (or "Ministresse des Affaires Amoureuses" in French), who recommends she does exactly that. This character is a member of the fictional Mouvement de Libération de la Négresse (MLN or "Movement for the Liberation of the Negress") whose platform encourages Afro-Caribbean women to "surveiller [leur homme], d'appliquer à la lettre ce que nos bonnes mamans nous ont enseigné. Faire les poches de chaque veste, inspecter le fond du caleçon, ouvrir l'oeil et les narines" (watch their man, to follow to the letter what our mindful mothers had taught us. To empty the pockets of each jacket, inspect the underwear in and out, keep both eyes and nostrils open) (*DD*, 121) because, "[g]are à toi la femme noire si tu t'avises d'oublier l'histoire!" (beware of forgetting history, Black woman!) (*DD*, 123).

In effect, this not so liberating sororal community only incites Frida to fall back on the designated path, that of learned caution and distrust, just like Eric reverted to historical stereotyping of Afro-Caribbean manhood. Faced with such a restrictive destiny for the feminine self, Afro-Caribbean men, and the couple, Frida enacts her freedom by desiring to consume, to devour the devourers, those driven by a figurative predatory instinct like her mother or Eric. First, as regards the haunting mother figure, she is one who, following Célia Sadai's perhaps quite harsh analysis of the character, "colporte des prescriptions confuses sur la race, qui transmet l'ignorance et la léthargie politique" (spreads confusing ordering principles, conveys ignorance and political lethargy) (2009). Frida's mother's repressive code of conduct, of which she was herself a victim, triggers the protagonist's increasing frustration and predatory anger. "J'ai faim de maman, ferais bien rôtir son corps à la broche, en découperais volontiers chaque morceau" (I am hungry for mom, would do well to roast her and would gladly slice her up), Frida admits. "Que signifie le désir de manger sa mère, docteur?" (What does the desire to eat your mother mean, doctor?) (*DD*, 170). Here, the tyranny of the mother results in Frida's drive toward destruction.

In the case of her mother, Frida's murderous instinct never translates to action, but Eric, the treacherous lover, meets a different fate. In her murder of Eric, Frida situates her practice of freedom, the ultimate liberation she was originally seeking in the reconstruction of the Antillean couple. At the murder scene, "Frida se félicite de ce crime. Elle a tué. Vient de contrevenir à la loi du silence de toute une génération" (Frida is pleased with this crime. She has killed. Has just broken the code of silence of a whole generation) (*DD*, 33). She continues, "Tu peux être fière de ta fille, papa. Tu peux sourire à présent, à présent que je suis une femme libre" (You can be proud of your daughter, Papa. You can smile now, now that I have become a free woman) (*DD*, 34). Indeed, Frida can exist now that she has refused a formerly inescapable cyclical history. And ultimately, the irresolvable paradox of her freedom comes at the cost of her own life—an act of self-annihilation that she *chooses* for herself, perhaps for the first time, after everything else has failed.

Thinking with scholars Hanétha Vété-Congolo and Kaiama Glover, I consider, in this last section of my discussion of *D'eaux douces*, the ways in which Frida's murder and final act of self-annihilation can be read at the intersection of the individual and community, self-care and solidarity. It means to linger on self-liberation and healing of the self before looking for the collectively deserving political intent, placing (self-)care, in whichever form (perhaps in the shape, in fiction, of a gory murder and suicide) as an essential precursor to collective thinking. In her analysis of *D'eaux douces*, Vété-Congolo principally reads Frida's final actions for their revolutionary intent, as a means to break free from the historical determinism perverting the Afro-Caribbean couple and restoring community and solidarity. For Vété-Congolo, Frida's actions introduce the possibility of "termine[r] le cycle de l'impasse et inscri[re] sa contre-action dans l'ouverture de la proposition dans le sens où elle tend à montrer la voie" (terminating the dead-end cycle and inscribing her counter-action in the expansion of the proposition in the sense that she aims to open the way) (2015, 121–122)—in short, "un acte de solidarité avec la postérité" (an act of solidarity for posterity) (2015, 119). In line with Vété-Congolo, then, Frida's actions are subsumed within a collective agenda, presenting the murder of Eric and her own suicide (tellingly by shooting at her vagina, the physical and symbolic site of historical oppression and violence) as an individual sacrifice to repair the community. But wouldn't putting the community first turn Frida into another self-sacrificing female figure, another kind of *poto-mitan*—the role she was originally refusing by denying her matrilineal legacy?

In *A Regarded Self: Caribbean Womanhood and the Ethics of Disorderly Being* (2021), Kaiama Glover studies practices of freedom that prioritize self rather than communal focus. Through an analysis of morally ambivalent and politically unaligned female protagonists, Glover considers the practice of self-regard for its own sake in social contexts where women find themselves in situations of oppression, repression, and possibly violence. The ways in which self-care manifests in Glover's literary corpus can seem unsettling or frustrating because the kinds of disorderly women she considers to "'misbehave'" (2021, 33) are, according to Glover, "adamantly unrecoverable" (3). In short, Glover emphasizes these women's refusal of community—a concept she links to "masculinist writers and literary movements such as Édouard Glissant's *Antillanité* and Jean Bernabé, Patrick Chamoiseau, and Raphaël Confiant's *Créolité*, but also, importantly, to womanist discourses that privilege the self-sacrificing and powerful *poteau mitan*" (Thomas 2021, 146). As such, Glover articulates her own refusal to read these women through any lens other than their self-regard.

Interestingly, Frida is one who also refuses to conform to the repressive social codes she inherits from her women-focused communities. However, she concurrently seeks to build the foundations of an alternative community, as well as a new Antillean couple, through her relationship with Eric. Eventually though, the failure of Frida's strategy leads to a possibly morally reprehensible turn of events (the murder of Eric), from which emerges her self-liberation ("je suis une femme libre," I have become a free woman; *DD*, 34). In light of Frida's murderous act and final self-annihilation, what would it mean to prioritize the character's journey of self-expression and self-care before or even instead of calling for the "liberation of the Negress" (*DD*, 130)? Frida herself seems to be primarily concerned with the survival or rather rebirth of the community; she is in fact consumed by the project of repairing community all the way into the conclusion of *D'eaux douces*: "Je m'appelle FD et je viens de tuer. . . . C'est pour la bonne cause. Pour préserver l'espèce" (My name is FD, and I have just killed. . . . It's for a good cause. For the preservation of our species) (*DD*, 207). In a way, the narrative itself inherently deflects a prolonged focus on the individual in Frida's radical final actions, which is tellingly reflected in scholarly interpretations of the novel (see Vété-Congolo 2015, but also Francis 2017 and Persson 2017, among others).[8]

Yet, following Glover's logic, there would be potential value in practices of refusal that "simply" bring into focus "individual expressions of defiance" (12). And, indeed, in defiance of the restrictive expectations imposed by both her maternal (dictating her to take on the roles of "a good wife, a good mother, a good maid," 12–13) and sororal community (urging her to follow "to the letter" the teaching of their mindful mothers; *DD*, 121), Frida ultimately enacts her personal liberation through the murder-suicide, a "deviant" act of self-care. In fact, before she resolves to the murder-suicide, Frida observes, in a moment of self-diagnosis, that since she learned of Eric's infidelity she had been taking care of herself, yet with no hope of healing (*DD*, 184). Thinking about her own death, she admits, "J'ai le sentiment qu'il ne me reste qu'elle" (I have the feeling this is the only option I have left) (*DD*, 184). Healing, truly caring for herself is constrained by her living because living would mean falling back on patterns of oppressive caring. Thus, to care means not to "maintain" the self (in reference to Tronto and Fisher's definition of the term) but rather to refuse to continue a disciplining social order.[9]

In effect, Frida's gesture of care is unconventional, deviant, but let us not forget it takes place within a context of oppressive caregiving norms. My intent here is not to delink Frida's act of self-care from the community the character wishes to reinvent—at least, not completely. Rather, it is an invitation to let Frida linger a moment longer in her defiance and self-liberation, especially when the future of the community, of the "liberated Negress," is yet to be written out of *D'eaux douces*.[10]

In *La bonne histoire de Madeleine Démétrius* (2020), Martinican writer Gaël Octavia tells the story in the first person of a woman who clashes dramatically with the type of female characters that Kanor portrays—figures who are ultimately rejected by Frida in *D'eaux douces*.[11] Octavia's female narrator-protagonist is a writer who has left Martinique to settle in Paris. She is also a single mother, whose children Nina and Eunice, are born from two different fathers. She "ne luttai[t] guère pour les empêcher de partir" (hardly fought to stop them from leaving) (*BH*, 71) and now shares custody of her daughters with both fathers. She refuses to pass for a continuously strong woman and determined mother—she shares her emotional heartbreaks (*BH*, 84) and occasionally questions wanting to be a parent (*BH*, 95). This narrator-protagonist, who appears liberated from the gender and societal expectations that typically befall Caribbean women—particularly those contained and constrained by the archetype of the *poto-mitan*, the mother courage—also confesses that she continuously faces criticism from her older daughter, who "appelle de ses voeux une mère plus rassurante" (wishes for a more reassuring mother) (*BH*, 91). She struggles with feelings of shame, deeply rooted in the very social pressures she seeks to escape.

In *La bonne histoire*, the ordering codes governing women's social existence, both within and outside the domestic space, manifest in the relationships the female characters—across generations and between hexagonal France and Martinique—foster and disband, at times permanently, despite who they are or because of the facades they project to society. In my analysis of Octavia's novel, I am thus interested in the ripple effect on this intergenerational ecosystem of women resulting from the dismantling of "la bonne histoire"—the controlled narrative of Caribbean womanhood that the narrator-protagonist is tasked with writing. What story can be written? What forms of existence are available to women outside the trodden path toward the *poto-mitan*? In short, I argue that *La bonne histoire* picks up where *D'eaux douces* left off and left us.

The novel opens with a precursory declaration: "Mon amie Madeleine m'a demandé d'écrire son histoire" (My friend Madeleine has asked me to write her story) (*BH*, 9). The narrator-protagonist meets with her estranged high school friend, Madeleine, who is making a flying visit to Paris; Madeleine has told her that she wishes to tell her about "quelque chose qu'[elle a] vécu et [dont la narratrice] v[a] . . . faire un livre" (something she has experienced and which the narrator is going to make into a book) (*BH*, 10). Briefly, Madeleine's story is that, during her middle school years, she and her friend Cynthia met a military man who had just arrived from hexagonal France. The first time they saw him, the two adolescents were on their way to Cynthia's house on their lunch break and caught him masturbating in his car. The next few times they ran into him, he insisted they come over for a Coke, repeatedly asking for their forgiveness. Madeleine recounts that her friend eventually accepted his invitation. After that first visit, they would go again; and, based on Madeleine's version of the story, Cynthia would disappear into the military man's bedroom, leaving Madeleine behind to wait for her friend's return. And, "[c]'était ça [that was that]," Madeleine concludes (*BH*, 41).

This sanitized narrative reinforces a normative script of respectability for Madeleine, who hails from a high-class Martinican Mulatto family. In Afro-Caribbean contexts, respectability, as discussed by scholars like Jacques André (1987) and Stéphanie Mulot (2000, 2009), is linked to notions of "discrétion sexuelle, inhibition, moralité et fidélité" (sexual discretion, inhibition, righteousness, and faithfulness) (119).[12] This portrayal mirrors the self-image Madeleine has carefully cultivated, maintained, and sought to project over time. In this case, the flip side of maintaining respectability involves denigrating her friend Cynthia, whom Madeleine identifies as "un summum de perversité" (the epitome of depravity) (*BH*, 50), although the latter has no voice in the matter.

In line with the stereotypical *poto-mitan*, the pillar of the family and society, which sociologist Sabine Lamour defines as "a figure of indefatigable strength in adversity, self-denial, intuition, empathy, generosity, tenacity, courage, resourcefulness, and dedication" (2021, 139), Madeleine conforms to a scripted idea of womanhood. The narrator-protagonist recalls a visit she made to Madeleine shortly after the latter had moved in with her partner Loïc, recounting the transformation of her friend into "une maîtresse de maison digne d'une publicité des années 50" (a lady of the house suitable for an advertisement from the 1950s) (*BH*, 81). "J'avais alors observé le soin maniaque porté à toute chose, scruté le sourire artificiel et étonnament blanc. J'avais l'impression d'être face à un robot" (I then witnessed the obsessive care given to everything, scrutinized the artificial but surprisingly white smile. I had the feeling I was facing a robot) (*BH*, 81), the narrator-protagonist comments. As presented by Madeleine, the "right" or "good" story (in French the adjective tellingly means either one) the narrator-protagonist is entrusted to write is meant to maintain the carefully crafted and controlled fiction of her friend's invented self. After all, with Madeleine "tout se passait toujours bien, tout était sous contrôle" (everything always went smoothly, everything was under control) (*BH*, 78).

Yet, through a *mise en abyme* of the writing process, the narrator-protagonist is able to start questioning what is in fact "right," and what makes for a "good" story. Interestingly, the double meaning of the adjective in French gestures toward the possibility to tell *a* truth, one that might or rather should diverge from Madeleine's version in order to do *right* by the women who have suffered the impact of oppressive narratives, thus challenging the prevailing trope of strength and resilience. Reflecting on the story just relayed to her, the narrator-protagonist attempts to begin writing—only to experience writer's block. After writing the word "*folle*" (crazy) on the page, she struggles to write more and is struck by a profound lethargy (*BH*, 52). This moment of pause has important implications for the narrator-protagonist's relationship to the story she has been commissioned to write, particularly as regards the version she eventually documents. While the "main" document remains irrevocably thin—in total, the narrator-protagonist will have written, intermittently, three apparently unrelated words ("folle," "séisme," [earthquake], and "esclave" [enslaved]), more attention and sustained work is paid to the "fichiers annexes" (appendices) that "voient leur volume croître de jour en jour, prennent l'allure de journaux intimes anachroniques" (see their volume increase day by day, taking the shape of anachronistic diaries) (*BH*, 91). Interestingly, the activity of annexing, from the French word "*annexe*," implicates etymologically "that which is joined," meaning something which serves as a derivative expansion or supplement. In this case, the invariably choppy and disjointed stories appended to her narrative become a central metaphor for both the refusal of controlled and ordering storytelling practices as well as the difficulty of telling that which is not known or uncomfortable to confront. All of which leads to the narrator-protagonist's interrogation through fictional possibilities.

"Qui avait manipulé qui, en vérité? Qui avait utilisé qui? Qui était l'appât?" (In reality, who manipulated whom? Who used whom? Who was the bait?) (*BH*, 110), the narrator asks—in short, "Qui est Cynthia?" (Who is Cynthia?) (*BH*, 112). The questions that increasingly animate the narrator-protagonist interfere greatly with the writing process, eventually driving much of the narrative and subverting the version originally presented by Madeleine. For indeed, as the narrator-protagonist pushes against the general and restrictive terms imposed by Madeleine to define Cynthia—"Saint Lucienne. Provocante. Mauvaise élève. Bonne cuisinière" (Saint Lucian. Seductive. Bad student. Good cook) (*BH*, 113)—she shifts the focus from the authoritative and cohesive narrative to the missing, absent, or untold. Through this, we see the narrator-protagonist question whether there is more to the story told by Madeleine.

One possibility the narrator-protagonist considers is exclusion that results from racialization: she momentarily suggests, before erasing the words from the page, Madeleine's possible attempt to symbolically "[b]annir la négresse" (banish the Negress), Cynthia, through the telling of this story (*BH*, 121). Another interpretation is Madeleine's suppression of an unsanctioned desire, when she would have in fact secretly "envied," "admired" the relation between Cynthia and the military man (*BH*, 60). This way, the narrator-protagonist manipulates the perception and configuration of this three-person relationship, thereby denying Madeleine narrative authority and fictionalizing instead the voice of the other ("la *bonne histoire* avait pris forme et c'était l'histoire de Cynthia Chantelle Murray" (the right story was taking shape, and it was the story of Cynthia Chantelle Murray) (*BH*, 154).

For the narrator-protagonist, this eventually constitutes an act of betrayal of allegiance, for she affirms, "Je me sens autorisée à fouiller le passé, à tout assumer, y compris le risque d'écorner l'image de Madeleine. De donner à voir la dérive douce, discrète, de mon amie" (I give myself permission to dig into the past, to take responsibility for everything, including the risk of tarnishing Madeleine's image. To show the gentle, discreet drift of my friend) (*BH*, 76). Presented only with a reductive and superficial version of the story, the narrator-protagonist then boldly asks, "Mais encore?" (And what else?) (*BH*, 113). To challenge the oppressive constraints of respectability is to propose a state of fictional instability, "creat[ing] and search[ing] for images of Black womanhood that . . . posit new narratives that point to alternative directions" as scholar Régine Michelle Jean-Charles suggests in her essay "Getting around the Poto-mitan" (2021, 28). In *La bonne histoire* this means to quite literally trace back the story to tell: the narrator-protagonist and her daughters, following an intense internet search, manage to excavate the figuratively missing Cynthia. During a trip to the region of Languedoc, where Cynthia owns an inn and restaurant "La Table de Miss Cissy," the characters symbolically enter "le territoire de Cynthia" (Cynthia's territory) (*BH*, 128). Although they do not establish direct contact with Cynthia, this expedition into so far obstructed narrative possibilities later fuels the version of *la bonne histoire* the narrator-protagonist eventually publishes.

Completing her novel is thus for the narrator-protagonist a means to proclaim her own independence ("Je ne suis pas ton esclave, Madeleine Démétrius," I am not your slave, she declares to and for herself; *BH*, 157), both revealing repressive fictional frameworks as well as building narrative practices of liberation. This results, in the course of the narrative, in the progressive unbolting, physically and metaphorically, of disciplining social and gender figures such as the *poto-mitan*. A prime example of this is in the announcement of Madeleine's stroke—a narrative device that shows the character's reorientation from the *poto-mitan* uprightness to vulnerable horizontality: "ce corps autrefois infiniment plus énergique que le mien" (this body once infinitely more energetic than mine) now "contraint à l'immobilité" (forced to immobility) (*BH*, 178). This family tragedy also allows a shift in how Madame Démétrius, Madeleine's mother, is viewed—thus far fictionalized by the narrator-protagonist as a woman "autoritaire et sûre d'elle" (bossy and confident) "capable de tout, même de l'impossible" (capable of achieving everything, even the impossible), "[une] mèr[e] surpuissant[e]" (a superpowerful mother) (*BH*, 193), she is eventually allowed to show weakness. Unbolting therefore comes to signify the demise of identity as one and undividable—a notion which may certainly appear in line with Glissant's theorizing of rhizomatic thought[13] against the concept of a unique root-identity. This demise becomes all the more manifest through the disbandment of the "tout indivisible" (undividable whole) that the narrator-protagonist believed she formed alongside her four high school friends, including Madeleine, as well as Petite Christelle, Grande Christelle, and Jessica. But this is not to lament friend estrangement; rather, it is to reassert the possibility of expansive and more accepting narrative forms of existence for women in Caribbean texts.

    For indeed, telling *la bonne histoire* from the perspective of Cynthia offers the narrator-protagonist a means to negotiate anew the feeling of shame caused by her perceived dysfunctionality and inadequacy as regards gendered respectability. Delving into the past, she admits, "Ce que je découvre cette semaine, moi qui prétends assumer les échecs de ma vie de femme, c'est que j'ai honte de ma honte, de cette honte ancienne" (What I discover this week, although I claim to accept the failures of my life as a woman, is that I am ashamed of my shame, of this old shame) (*BH*, 94–95). For reclaiming liberated scripts of womanhood involves challenging deeply entrenched social and gender norms, which as such cannot be easily dismissed. In the essay "Peut-on être guadeloupéenne, potomitan et féministe?" Mulot notes, through a sociological study, the stability of the cultural archetype of the *poto-mitan* which, rooted in the imagery of the Mulâtresse Solitude (in a Guadeloupean context), remains central in women's conversations either as "model" (model) or "repoussoir" (deterrent) (2021, 126).[14] As the *poto-mitan* elicits ambivalence from the women she interviewed, Mulot observes that consequently women tend to neglect gender-related issues, privileging instead class struggle and nationalistic aspirations (124). Given the marginalization of women's self-expression, it is unsurprising that Octavia's narrator-protagonist has yet to come to terms with a version of womanhood that is not the *poto-mitan*.

In describing her life as a woman and mother, the narrator-protagonist recounts with complete transparency her moments of frailty and vulnerability; for example, when she feels "trop lasse . . . pour chercher à reprendre les rênes de la maisonnée, à exercer un quelconque contrôle sur leurs allées et venues, sur leurs activités" (too tired to try to take back control of the household, to watch over their [Nina and Eunice's] comings and goings and activities) (*BH*, 176). The role of the "maîtresse de maison hors-pair" (unsurpassed lady of the house), that of Madeleine, is not one she aspires to reproduce. Rather, she acknowledges the cracks in the ceiling and the dilapidated state of her own house, both in its physical and metaphorical dimensions. All of these have in fact become defining aspects of her character ("Je suis une maison décrépite," I am a decrepit house, the narrator-protagonist thinks to herself; *BH*, 176).

From the perspective of Nina, her older daughter, the narrator-protagonist's vulnerability appears to be a weakness, thereby justifying Nina assuming control over their household, commanding while also infantilizing her mother. For instance, after announcing the visit of Madeleine's husband, Loïc, for dinner following his wife's accident, the narrator-protagonist recounts that Nina and Eunice took the initiative of doing the shopping and preparing the meal. As she describes herself, "Fébrile, je me joins à mes filles, cheffe et petit marmiton s'affairant à la cuisine, prête à peler, ébouillanter, rissoler à leurs côtés, mais Nina m'ôte des mains couteau et planche à découper comme si j'étais une enfant sur le point de se blesser. . . . 'Va plutôt t'occuper de toi-même!'" (Feverish, I join my daughters, chef and little kitchen hand busy in the kitchen, ready to peel, boil, brown alongside them, but Nina takes the knife and cutting board from my hands as if I were a child about to hurt herself. . . . "Go take care of yourself instead!") (*BH*, 180). The narrator-protagonist's relinquishing of control, of this "comédie de l'autorité" (show of authority) between mother and daughter, compels Nina to assume the responsibility of protecting and taking care of her mother (*BH*, 129). In doing so, the character demonstrates what she considers strength when she sees it lacking, stepping into the role of the "better" mother—"plus exigeante, plus rigide, plus directive et plus efficace" (more demanding, strict, bossy, and efficient)—she wishes she had had (*BH*, 175).

In light of this, the narrator-protagonist perceives in Nina an excessive strictness, which she fears might transform her into "[une] inconnue au coeur sec, [une] statue sans mollesse ni tendresse" (a stranger with a cold heart, a statue lacking softness or kindness) (*BH*, 168), but she remains hesitant to fully reveal herself to her daughters, fearing their judgment and contempt. For this unrestrained visibility, while marking her own self-definition, would also render her all the more vulnerable.

Tell them about how you're never really a whole person if you remain silent, because there's always that one little piece inside you that wants to be spoken out, and if you keep ignoring it, it gets madder and madder and hotter and hotter, and if you don't speak it out one day it will just up and punch you in the mouth from the inside. (Lorde [1984] 2007, 42)

These are the words of Audre Lorde's daughter to her mother, as quoted in the essay "The Transformation of Silence into Language and Action." Through this, Lorde challenges herself, and us, to overcome this "fear of visibility" because doing so would mean to be seen and heard for what we are. In *La bonne histoire*, there is a clear transition from the "secret" appendices where the narrator-protagonist cautiously records private anecdotes, fearing "qu'elles [Nina et Eunice] lisent par-dessus [son] épaule" (they read over [her] shoulder) (*BH*, 94), to the publication of the story that was not meant to be told, one for which she elicited and came to grips with her shame. To write the character of Cynthia, the narrator-protagonist confesses, "je devrais l'autoriser à aller puiser en moi, à se saisir de ma honte" (I should allow her to dig deep inside of me, to take hold of my shame) (*BH*, 154), thereby rendering visible her vulnerability while reversing (self-)imposed silencing in a transformative gesture of self-affirmation.

In considering the pivotal role of reclamation of vulnerability in *La bonne histoire*, I think now with scholar Fabienne Brugère about the relationship between caring and the experience of vulnerability. It means highlighting how caring relationships take new shape through the unmaking of the taboo of vulnerability in Afro-Caribbean contexts. In *Le sexe de la sollicitude* (2008), Brugère links practices of care with women, invoking "un imaginaire de mère bienveillante et d'épouse attentive" (an imagination of a kind mother and attentive wife) (11) that supports the gender-specific task of managing vulnerability. Yet Brugère also reminds us, "Il importe de ne pas oublier que les sujets qui exercent la sollicitude et prennent soin des humains en situation de vulnérabilité sont eux-mêmes des êtres vulnérables" (It is important to not forget that the individuals who show concern and care for human beings in vulnerable situations are themselves vulnerable) (14). Indispensable to the maintenance of the family and the household, the *potomitan* is clearly one who gives care, but the focus is on "their strength and ability to overcome," Jean-Charles also notes (2021, 18). The glorification and naturalization of such characteristics thus does not call for recognition of vulnerability following Brugère. One that, conversely, the narrator-protagonist strives for as she asserts her own self aside from the fictionalization of women's resilience and strength.

We also see how the narrator-protagonist's gradual acceptance of vulnerability shifts her interactions with the women and girls around her. Initially, at times signaling her vulnerable self through inner speech, she contains it within for fear of being reprimanded or judged by Nina. This leaves her faced with an internal dilemma: "N'ai-je pas à coeur de me montrer telle quelle, sans chercher à paraitre plus forte ou plus exemplaire . . . ?" (Don't I want to show myself as I am, without trying to appear stronger or more exemplary?) (*BH*, 91). At other times, she awkwardly attempts to undermine her daughter's self-appointed authority. The narrator-protagonist recalls a moment when, upon hearing Nina return home, she thought about hiding the pâté jar to avoid upsetting her daughter, a fervent vegan, but eventually decided not to. "Me soumettre à la tyrannie de ma fille," she concedes, "n'a rien de bon ni pour moi ni pour elle" (Giving in to my daughter's tyranny does nothing good for me or her) (*BH*, 61). For, as Brugère suggests, is "reconnaître cette vulnérabilité" (to recognize this vulnerability)—even if manifested solely through a little weakness for pâté—not to "savoir s'en préoccuper" (know how to take care of it) (2008, 31)? But perhaps this is not immediately the case if we consider Nina's ensuing diatribe against her mother's perceived irresponsibility. Over the course of the narrative though, Nina demonstrates more frequently, yet shyly, the vulnerability, the softness that the narrator-protagonist wishes her to show.

Toward the end of the novel, after the publication of the writer-narrator's *La bonne histoire* and during the family's trip to

Martinique, Nina reveals to her mother she has been corresponding with Cynthia since they went to Languedoc, wanting to know more about being a chef. "J'observe, amusée, ma fille qui se livre sans retenue" (I pleasantly observe my daughter confiding in me unrestrainedly), the narrator-protagonist says (*BH*, 240), but "Nina finit par s'apercevoir que je la scrute. Son visage retrouve une certaine dureté, comme si elle claquait le volet d'une fenêtre à laquelle je l'avais épiée à son insu" (Nina ends up noticing that I'm scrutinizing her. Her expression hardens again, as if she were slamming the shutter of a window through which I had spied on her without her knowledge). By briefly letting herself be seen, the character's usual display of authority that the inherited *poto-mitan* archetype supports appears brittle. This visibility, which makes her vulnerable, also makes space for attention and a softer way of caring, both from her mother but also for herself.

Thus, this means to reinvent the relations that organize caring, doing away with the master narrative of the *poto-mitan* that maintains an archetype of sacrificial, tough care. It is the letting go of such fantasized and idealized "omnipotence of women" (Lamour 2021, 138) that allows other stories of the self to be told, as we see for example with Nina's cautious steps toward self-expression. More generally, the telling of "*la bonne histoire*" is what liberates, as characters let their truths be seen and see others anew. The novel's epilogue in Martinique verifies this explicitly. While she is there to see Madeleine at the hospital, the narrator-protagonist also attempts to reconnect with the other former members of the disbanded "undividable whole." She meets with Grande Christelle, whom the narrator-protagonist identifies originally as a "ravèt lègliz" in Kreyòl (a very devoted churchwoman). During the conversation, Grande Christelle challenges the narrator-protagonist's view of her and their former high school friends, exposing the illusion of respectability that had distorted her understanding of their distinct realities. "La Madeleine du lycée. La plus sage d'entre nous. Elle n'est plus comme ça" (High school's Madeleine. The most well-behaved among us. She is no longer like that), Grande

Christelle announces abruptly. She continues, telling the narrator-protagonist about the secrets Madeleine confided in her, particularly as regards the affairs and numerous lovers she had over the years. This final revelation is an additional disruption to the narrative the narrator-protagonist had fabricated, which not only had stood as an obstacle to the expression of their respective voices and experiences but also had fueled her own feeling of shame.

Similarly, earlier in *La bonne histoire*, the narrator-protagonist, reflecting on the disbandment of the "undividable whole," convinces herself that their diverging paths in adulthood caused them to drift apart—a testament, one may think, to the inevitable divide that arises when one "misbehaves," which means here to stray from societal norms of womanhood. However, in the end, Grande Charlotte points instead to the perceived social inadequacy of those who stayed behind, this time under the influence of their fabricated truth about their friend: "'On t'imaginait dans ta vie parisienne. On te savait dans ton cercle d'artistes, avec ton homme artiste'" ("'We imagined you living the Parisian life. We knew you were surrounding yourself with artists, and your artist boyfriend'") (*BH*, 253). These conflicted perspectives all serve a similar purpose, to become aware of preconceived notions and biases and pay attention to the once (self-)neglected selves that exhort to be seen and heard. What *La bonne histoire* does for us then is to put forward an avenue for reconciliation: exploring the self outside the prescriptive *poto-mitan* model allows these women and girls to reclaim visibility and care for themselves and each other.

The potential for reconciliation might thus be seen in the gesture depicted in the last pages of the novel between Madame Démétrius and Rosalie, the housekeeper with whom Monsieur Démétrius was having an affair. "Madame Démétrius pose une main affectueuse sur l'épaule de Rosalie, qui lui sourit en retour" (Madame Démétrius places an affectionate hand on Rosalie's shoulder, who smiles back at her) (*BH*, 262). In this gentle gesture, a renewed attention to the quiet visibilities that are being formed outside hierarchies of gendered respectability becomes manifest.

I started the second section of this chapter mentioning the possibility to read *D'eaux douces* and *La bonne histoire* in sequence because they both grapple with the *poto-mitan* cultural archetype; they both refuse it but go about this very differently. Both Kanor and Octavia incorporate this prescriptive model of Afro-Caribbean womanhood into fiction to allow for its diagnosis, manipulation, and potential undoing while also interrogating the possibilities and limitations in representing Caribbean women and girls in fiction. In writing the violent and radical murder-suicide in *D'eaux douces*, Kanor reminds us that caring is deeply rooted in colonial oppression and the gendered legacy of slavery, and she questions the possibility of retrieval of self. Frida's undoing of self markedly introduces us to unscripted, perhaps more hopeful territories of womanhood, but the attention we, as readers, can pay to Frida is also key to restoring her originally denied selfhood. This restoration of self is precisely what Octavia articulates in *La bonne histoire* by allowing female characters to not go by the script; unlike Kanor's Frida, Octavia's women achieve visibility by obliterating the fiction of the *poto-mitan* rather than their own selves. As such, *La bonne histoire* reenergizes the potential of caring to shape practices of attention to both the liberated self and others. Such caring could also have reclaimed Frida's self-expression.

Coda

This book was an invitation to interrogate our understandings of care, the ways it manifests itself historically and the caring relationships that may take shape when delinked from the forms of inequality and domination instituted under colonial rule. Throughout, I have discussed the decolonial reflections on care that originate from the French Caribbean and are found in French Caribbean texts (visual and written) and contexts that have been marked by this historical legacy. To conclude this conversation, I turn to Gisèle Pineau once again, but this time to consider the *récit* (narrative) *Folie, aller simple: Journée ordinaire d'une infirmière* (Madness, a one-way ticket: an ordinary day in the life of a nurse, 2010; hereafter *FAS*). Pineau's autobiographical reflections in *Folie, aller simple* highlight her own experiences working as a psychiatric nurse between Guadeloupe and the Paris region. Pineau recounts that she worked for twenty years at the Saint Claude psychiatric hospital in Guadeloupe, between the years 1980 and 2000, but at the time she wrote her récit she had moved back to the Paris region and was working at the Esquirol de Saint-Maurice hospital.

Quite notably, in the introduction to the conference proceedings "Souci d'autrui, soin, écriture" (2022), scholars Andrea Oberhuber and Alexandre Gefen identify Pineau's oeuvre as the prime example of "un dispositif d'aide, voire un médicament" (an assistive device, some sort of medication even).[1] In Pineau's work, the figures of the writer and nurse converge, drawing writing closer to an act of care, a care practice, while also emphasizing the reparative and restorative work involved in nursing. In fact, regarding her own practice Pineau writes in *Folie, aller simple* that she is both a writer and a nurse, highlighting the commonality between these professions in the focused attention ("une attention toute particulière," a specific type of attention; *FAS*, 150) they both require.

"Les mots que les infirmiers choisissent sont des instruments de soin" (The words nurses choose are care instruments), Pineau writes, considering more specifically the way words may manifest caring relationships, encouraging us to interrogate what caring attitudes may be reflected in, if not even interlaced with, the spoken and written word (*FAS*, 175). What makes words gestures of care? How can words carve out a caring space? I propose in this final reflection to explore words, and more particularly literature, as a place that embodies *care*ful attention and thus actively participates in shaping, maintaining, or restoring empathy, shared vulnerability, interdependency, and attentiveness to the self, others, and the world we live in. Turning to Pineau's text, I interrogate the intersection of caring and writing/words from a place—the psychiatric hospital—historically conceptualized as being outside and apart from our world since the early modern period in Europe.

In his study *History of Madness* (2013), Michel Foucault claims that madness, dating back to at least the mid-seventeenth century, became associated with confinement—also termed, after Foucault, the "grand renfermement" (great internment): the introduction of an enclosed and isolating space to segregate those deemed socially deviant from the rest of society. The space that Foucault describes is one that reduces pathologized individuals to silence and invisibility, thus entrapping them in a state of social nonexistence (or "non-être"—nonbeing—to use Foucault's terminology). In the introduction to their edited volume *Quand la folie parle* (When madness speaks; 2014), scholars Gillian Ni Cheallaigh, Laura Jackson, and Siobhán McIlvanney suggest contrastingly that against the entrapment of madness and the asylum there is a possibility to "learn of, and from, the human experiences, truths and tragedies that exist at the heart of humanity under the guise of madness" (2).

In fact, Pineau immediately undoes symbolically the walls of the psychiatric hospital when readers encounter this space in the narrative's opening paragraph—the nurse receives news of the suicide of a patient, "Mademoiselle Sophie R.," and answers questions from the police as Sophie's body is recovered from the metro train tracks.[2] The writer insists on a persistent outside/inside spatial boundary—she stands on the side of the care workers, the "porteurs de clés" (the key-bearers), "ceux qui entrent et sortent de l'hôpital en toute liberté" (those who can enter and leave the hospital quite freely)—but the psychiatric hospital nonetheless becomes a space of experimentation of caring (*FAS*, 16). Caring, in this context, somehow moves away from the role of the nurse as care worker, as the one who tends to her patients in the medical sense of the term.

In sum, caring is not so much thematic (i.e., a focus on health care workers or patients, for example, or a story that takes place in a retirement home or a hospital) than it is about the way Pineau writes about and reflects on her activity. In practice, the writer-nurse seeks to emancipate herself from the patient-nurse relationship established in an institutional framework and to develop instead a caring attitude despite the codification of the practice of nursing and an overwhelming workload. First, as part of the profession's strict regulation, Pineau notes the obligation for "une professionnelle de la santé" (a health care provider) to maintain a degree of emotional distance, to not "se laisser dominer par [s]es émotions" (be controlled by one's emotions) (*FAS*, 85). From the sole perspective of a French health system which appears rigid, Pineau's nursing activity is thus held back by restraint as health professionals are to be neither fully outside nor inside the psychiatric hospital.

Second, Pineau insists on the existence of an organizational hierarchy, further solidifying a boundary between patients and health professionals, which is linked to wearing a white coat inside the hospital. "Porter une blouse blanche dans une unité de soins psychiatriques" (Wearing a white coat in a psychiatric ward), Pineau explains, "ce n'est pas seulement afficher une autorité ou un pouvoir, c'est s'exposer à tous les maux, se poser en référent des lieux, gardien du temple, ange de la guérison, missionnaire en sacerdoce" (it is not only displaying authority or power, it also means exposing oneself to all aches, acting like the go-to person, a guardian of the temple, an angel of healing, a missionary in the priesthood) (*FAS*, 57). Here also, the nurse's seeming authority is quickly weighed down under the enumeration of the many hats they wear. Nursing care, Pineau adds, takes on numerous aspects, including "plombier, mécanicien, buraliste, assistante sociale, couturière, esthéticienne, astrologue, teinturière, Miss Météo, cuisinier en chef, confesseur, sexologue, comique troupier, animateur de karaoké [etc.]" (plumber, mechanic, shop clerk, social worker, couturier, beautician, astrologist, dry cleaner, weather presenter, cook, confessor, sexologist, comic, karaoke host, etc.) (*FAS*, 57). In addition to direct patient care responsibilities, these accumulated informal tasks highlight the expansive role nurses play within the psychiatric hospital.

While this gives insight into what exists beyond the initially strict vertical structure of the institution—which, according to Pineau, emphasizes maintaining emotional and physical distance from patients—it also alerts readers to the many responsibilities that nurses face. Indeed, the nurse portrayed by Pineau is involved in every aspect of ordinary life and needs, but this continuous demand, depicted as a "deflagration," can be overwhelming and taxing: the writer-nurse has the impression that she is "un pot de confiture attaqué par un essaim d'abeilles voraces" (a jar of jam attacked by a swarm of bees) (*FAS*, 57). This environment may significantly impact nurses' capacity to provide care to patients.

By emphasizing this avalanche of tasks, Pineau thus also alerts readers to the endangerment of nurses' well-being. Following the death of Sophie, Pineau and her shift partner, Noémie, are described as being "ébranlées, à moitié ramollies" (shaken, half numb) (*FAS*, 112). In the narrative, Sophie becomes a leitmotiv, a recurring ghostly presence who keeps reappearing at different moments of Pineau's workday. For example, when the writer-nurse recounts the ritualized moment of medication administration and the different patient profiles, especially the "contestaires routiniers" (those who routinely refuse medication), she remembers Sophie: "Elle n'a jamais accepté ces fameuses gouttes et comprimés" (She never willingly took these infamous drops and pills) (90). On a different occasion, a patient calls out to Pineau asking, "'Alors, infirmière! On la fait, cette partie de petits chevaux?'" ("Hey, nurse! When are we playing Ludo?"); the writer-nurse recalls, "Sophie aimait bien jouer aux petits chevaux, au Mikado, au Scrabble aussi" (Sophie liked playing Ludo, Mikado, and Scrabble) (63).

Pineau's inner monologue admonishes herself to remain a composed, comforting, and cheerful presence in troubled times: these verbs are all in the infinite form—"apaiser, rassurer, sentir, dérider, désamorcer, écouter, encore et encore" (pacifying, reassuring, feeling, cheering up, defusing, listening, again and again)—to denote necessity or obligation (58). But the writer-nurse is in fact battling her own emotional and physical frailty. There is a constant juxtaposition between what she should do and her troubled state after the news of Sophie's suicide. "Non, je ne vais pas faire une tête d'enterrement parce que Sophie est morte en début d'après-midi" (No, I will not look dispirited because Sophie died early this afternoon), the writer-nurse admonishes herself. "Non, je ne vais pas ajouter de l'angoisse à la pesanteur ambiante. Je vais chasser une à une les terribles images qui m'assaillent" (No, I will not add anxiety to the heaviness of the atmosphere. I will chase away one by one the terrible images that assail me) (*FAS*, 83). The ritualized behavior and actions she seeks to maintain are therefore constantly confronted with sporadic bouts of confusion, disorder, and distress, her own and that of others. In the final section of the récit, Pineau describes herself and Noémie as "deux somnambules" (two sleepwalkers) (*FAS*, 178) after having endured the physical and emotional toll of their workday—that is, everything that happens once one breaks through the silence of a seemingly structured and ritualized work environment.

A caring attitude unfolds as Pineau redirects attention on otherwise too often silenced but shared (as in the case of the writer-nurse and her shift partner Noémie) vulnerabilities and repressed emotions. Care writing, or writing as care, is situated in the framework of perception the narrative introduces, one that takes into account the particular relations of proximity and forms of attention that take shape within this "microsociété de la marge" (microsociety on the margins) (*FAS*, 60) that the psychiatric hospital represents, starting with the figure of the nurse that we have just discussed. Moreover, as the writer-nurse tells about the individuals she encounters and reminisces about others, Pineau attempts to reverse the distance from others and the subsequent invisibility. Similar to the work of undoing the codified imaginary that enshrouds the nurse figure, the writer-nurse seeks to bring visibility and attentive listening to her everyday interactions with patients. As Gefen and Oberhuber interrogate the possibility for "une littérature du *care*" (caring literature) to "prioriser . . . l'horizontalité des relations humaines plutôt que la verticalité et des structures de pouvoir hégémoniales" (prioritize . . . horizontality of human relations over verticality and hegemonic power structures), Pineau explores instances where relationships with others, regardless of their status (patient or care worker) within the hospital, can be (re-)created or restored.

One initial action involves disrupting how the nurse's presence is usually perceived by patients. This demands delineating a space outside a regimented hospital routine where the nurse can become ordinary. The return to everyday life occurs in the lulls ("ces moments creux d'après-goûter et d'avant-dîner" [These quiet moments after the 4pm snack and before dinner]; *FAS*, 135), characterized by the sudden indistinctness of those sharing the same space, thus allowing their relationships to be reimagined. The courtyard (referred to as "la cour" in French; *FAS*, 135), where nurses can join the patients when the hustle and bustle finally subsides, serves as both a physical and symbolic refuge. There, patients and care workers alike can quite literally step outside and shape their own interiority, their own way of being with others, free from a prescriptive and medicalized hospital interior. In the stillness of the hospital's courtyard, focus is reoriented on developing an ordinary presence to the self and others, as well as an attention to the seemingly mundane.

L'heure est à la langueur, à l'attente, une sorte d'entracte. On se satisfait des petits riens qui viennent effriter les heures. Dans ce moratoire, il n'y a pas d'enjeux, pas de spectacle, pas de prise de pouvoir, pas de démonstration. On cause ou pas. . . . On dit "Bah!" Et puis on soupire. . . . On grille une cigarette. . . . Et puis on regarde se consumer une allumette. On pousse de la pointe du pied un caillou, un mégot. (*FAS*, 135)

It is time for languor and waiting. A sort of intermission. We are satisfied with the little things that chip away at the hours. During this momentary respite, there are no issues, no performance, no takeover, no demonstration. We talk or not. . . . We say, "Oh well!" And then we sigh. . . . We smoke a cigarette. . . . And then we watch a match burn. We push a stone, or a cigarette butt, with the tip of the foot.

The actions described, as well as the rhythm of sentences, mark a slowness that is in stark contrast with the fast pace of hospital routine described previously. In introducing slowness, almost contemplation, the individual and the surroundings are *seen* differently. There, the nurse becomes "une personne ordinaire parmi des gens ordinaires" (an ordinary person among ordinary people) (*FAS*, 136). Already then, this type of writing, which Gefen terms a "littérature attentionnelle" (literature cultivating attention) in his anthological work *Réparer le monde: La littérature française face au XXIe siècle*, inaugurates a space of recuperation and reinvention of social relations, instructing us to slow down to notice the ordinary, to see what may otherwise remain unknown, overlooked, or disregarded. Pineau's writing style thus demonstrates her attempt to dismantle potential barriers, such as identities (i.e., the nurse/patient dyad) and specific locations (i.e., the psychiatric hospital) in narrating her experiences with patients and coworkers. The writer-nurse's literary practice is what shapes the expression of caring, and as such constitutes a prime experimentation with care writing, which somewhat resembles "narrative medicine."

The field of narrative medicine originated in the United States in the early 2000s at the instigation of physician Rita Charon (2001). Conceived as a way "to bridge the divides that separate the physician from the patient, the self, colleagues, and society" (2001, 1901), narrative medicine is defined by Charon in her introductory essay "Narrative Medicine: A Model for Empathy, Reflection, Profession, and Trust" as the development of a narrative competence in medicine as a means to nourish empathy and reflective engagement. In the context of the patient–physician relationship that Charon considers, physicians with narrative competence can build and maintain personal connections with their patients, as they have the ability to "absorb, interpret, and respond to stories" of others (2001, 1897). The narrative dimensions of caregiving that Charon supports in the case of medical practice can thus be easily enough transposed to the larger sphere of health care professionals to include, for example, nurse practitioners like Pineau. In fact, Pineau, in her capacity as both a nurse and a writer, provides us with a firsthand look at the application of caregiving with narrative competence as she shares her experiences at the psychiatric hospital. Her writing thus becomes an exercise in narrative medicine, the site of experimentation of what care and attention given to the particular look like, and where the narrative tools to acknowledge and respond to the stories of others are tested out.

Perhaps quite paradoxically, the narrative qualities of Pineau's caring practice are most evident in the untold stories. These narratives not only bring to light the invisibilized care work performed by the nurses and their daily challenges, but also incite to pay particular attention to those who at times wish to remain invisible.[3] "Toujours penser à ces patients qui deviennent transparents, finissent par se fondre dans le décor, se diluer dans le groupe" (Always think of these patients who become transparent, end up fading into the background, taking a back seat) the writer-nurse reminds herself while also cautioning us, "Toujours s'inquiéter d'untel qui ne réclame rien et s'efface derrière ceux qui donnent de la voix. Toujours accorder une écoute à ceux qui se font oublier, qui ne posent pas de problème" (Always worry about someone who never asks for anything and effaces themselves behind those who raise their voice. Always attach importance to those who wish to be forgotten, who don't cause any problems) (*FAS*, 74). Silence is thus what triggers the urge to preserve visibility.

When the writer-nurse tries to reveal what is already there but is not always seen or heard, a caring attitude takes shape through writing as her narrative affirms that they are in fact seen, acknowledged, and remembered. Clearly Pineau's text integrates numerous voices and subjectivities that come to be known by the reader. In the section anticipatedly titled "Je me souviens d'Adrien" (I remember Adrien), the writer-nurse juxtaposes repeatedly over a few paragraphs the anaphora "Je me souviens" (I remember) followed by the name of a former patient with gestures of denial, dismissal, or neglect. For example, Pineau "[s]e souvien[t] d'Inès et de ses TOC" (remembers Inès and her obsessive-compulsive disorder); "sa mère n'en pouvait plus et lui avait trouvé un studio" (her mother could not stand it anymore and had found her a studio apartment) (*FAS*, 189), which highlights how family members may feel burdened by caregiving. In Pineau's recounting of names and memories, rejection of madness by the wider society for what has become an unwanted disturbance is also evidenced. One paragraph begins with Pineau recalling Gaspard ("Je me souviens de Gaspard," I remember Gaspard) and concludes with "pendant son hospitalisation, les locataires et propriétaires de l'immeuble avaient signé une pétition et demandé l'expulsion de Gaspard et son frère" (during Gaspard's hospital stay, the tenants and owners of the building where he lived with his brother had signed a petition asking for their eviction) (*FAS*, 189). I want to emphasize that my intention here is in no way to criticize the lack of attention or failure to care adequately. Instead, I wish to underline the potential to recover attention and how it manifests in literature. This is particularly significant when this capacity for attention is tested in daily life situations, whether in the demanding context of nursing, or when family members or relatives refuse or are unable to provide care, or when bystanders choose disengagement or denial over attentiveness.

In this respect, Pineau's narrative provides a vital interrogation of what scholars Maïté Snauwaert and Dominique Hétu (2018) term "*care* du littéraire" (caring literature) in their introduction to the special issue "Poétiques et imaginaires du *care*," as Pineau's writing becomes a highly reflexive space where care is not only tested but also amplified. Of the five aspects they identify as pertinent to caring literature, two are particularly useful to us. One of those aspects—"la capacité des phrases à attirer notre attention et faire lumière sur ce qui est autrement invisible, inconnu, négligé" (the capacity of sentences to attract our attention and illuminate what might otherwise go unnoticed, invisible, remain unknown, or be overlooked)—we can see, for example, in Pineau's use of anaphora, the redundancy consolidating attention. Although it is beneficial for us to see how this capacity is effectively realized, *Folie, aller simple* also allows us to engage with caring as a learned practice, often put to the test and constantly developing.

In the case of Pineau, the evolution of her caring practice seems to start after she learns a very practical skill, that of administering injections in the context of a traumatic incident. Pineau specifically recounts her experience with her first patient, "Madame X," which left her in a state of devastation ("effondrée" in French; *FAS*, 133). Madame X, Pineau recalls, vehemently opposed the nurse administering the injection, screaming racial slurs at her (*FAS*, 133). Since then, Pineau writes, she "n'[a] cessé d'apprendre" (never ceased to learn) (*FAS*, 130)—converting what might have profoundly affected her at the start of her career into a mere unpleasantness. "*J'ai appris* à prendre des coups, à recevoir des jurons de toute facture, à supporter la folie ordinaire, son cortège de désagréments" (I learned to take a blow, to be called many names, to endure ordinary madness, and its share of inconvenience), Pineau writes (*FAS*, 131). She adds, "*J'ai appris* la patience et l'humilité, la rigueur et l'observation, la compassion et l'écoute silencieuse" (I learned to be patient and humble, rigorous and observing, compassionate and quietly attentive) (*FAS*, 130, emphases mine). Certainly, this new deployment of anaphoric repetition speaks to the progressive and learned attitude recentering caring for others, but it is one that also incites us perhaps to question the limits and impact of such a burden of attention.

For it is true that Pineau delivers a "warts-and-all narrative," as scholar Gillian Ni Cheallaigh et al. describe it—one "that unflinchingly chronicles the stresses, challenges (emotional and physical) and true human reality of the daily experience of the nurse within the asylum" (2014, 92). What then warrants Pineau's own survival and self-preservation? What serves to absorb her own vulnerability? Turning again to Snauwaert and Hétu (2018), we might see the second aspect of caring literature that they identify—"la pratique littéraire" (literary practice) as its own "pratique du soin, un mode d'accès vers un aller-mieux personnel ou vers un vivre-ensemble" (care practice, a way to achieve personal well-being or a sense of togetherness)—as a way to further explore the potential of narrative writing for recovery of the self. Pineau in fact actively anticipates our inquiry, observing that "l'écriture [l']a sauvée du pire" (writing saved her from the worst) for if "[elle] n'avai[t] pas eu l'écriture, [elle] aurai[t] pu [elle]-même être atteinte d'une 'affection psychiatrique'" (she had not had writing, she could have herself suffered from a "mental health condition") (*FAS*, 151). Similar to the garden space within the psychiatric hospital experienced as a refuge physically and symbolically, writing serves as Pineau's own escape from an at times overwhelming day-to-day existence; writing provides a way to momentarily move away from the well-trodden path. Interestingly in *Folie, aller simple*, Pineau explores the etymological and symbolic relationship between writing and losing one's mind (*délirer* in French). First, etymologically, the French word "délirer" derives from the term *delirare* in Latin, which means "to go off the furrow," to derail.[4] Symbolically then, Pineau asks, "Est-ce qu'écrire est une manière élégante et transversale de délirer?" (Does writing elegantly intersect with madness?) (*FAS*, 153). It is with this way of seeing the act of writing that the latter may enable a diversion off the path of madness. Consequently, to conceive of writing as a form of diversion accentuates the possibility for the practice of writing to create a healing space for recovery—one that Pineau may not find elsewhere.

But recognizing the essential role of the writer-nurse's inner life and imagination in maintaining her sanity also brings attention to the potential consequences of an impossible withdrawal from a chaotic world that could drive people mad. In an interview with scholar Valérie Loichot, Pineau remarked, "I write because writing is as vital as eating and drinking. If I don't write every day, I feel that my day is ruined. I don't feel good. I feel awful" (2007, 334). Compared to a basic need, writing ensures survival. The back and forth between the reality of everyday life and the world of fiction, as well as between Pineau-the-writer and Pineau-the-nurse, has its own therapeutic qualities because it allows Pineau to cope with and heal from the traumas of her individual history. However, as scholar Bonnie Thomas reminds us in her analysis of *Folie, aller simple*, Pineau's narrative also "reveals the often fragile separation that exists between madness and 'normality'" (2017, 71) as the writer places herself as well as her readers in close proximity with the eventuality of madness. In fact, returning to the imagery of the garden as a place of refuge in order to question it, Pineau suggests that "le gentil jardinet" (the sweet little garden) may one day change into "une forêt" (a forest) where "les tiges volubiles prolifèrent et menacent de vous étrangler" (the creeping stems proliferate and threaten to strangle you) (*FAS*, 155). As Thomas justly notes in her reading of this passage, "the threat of a garden growing out of control is ever present" (2017, 74), with the result of always narrowing more "the distance or separation between them [the nurses] [us] and the patient" (Ni Cheallaigh, Jackson, and McIlvanney 2014, 91).

This way, much of Pineau's narrative interrogates the borders of madness, inviting us to consider instead the ordinariness of mental disorders in our lived experiences and personal encounters as well as those of individuals around us. The mad Other thus breaches the walls of the psychiatric hospital to inhabit the everyday and pushes all the way into the private sphere. For example, in recounting a conversation with Francky, a Guadeloupean friend and candidate for the nursing entrance examination, Pineau recalls that as Francky listed different patient profiles in a psychiatric hospital, her thoughts were immediately filled with images of corresponding family members. When hearing about "des bonnes dames qui ont perdu la parole" (the kind women who have lost the ability to speak), Pineau is, for instance, reminded of her own maternal aunt, Gisèle; after the premature death of her young husband, Gisèle stopped eating, drinking, and speaking and died at the age of twenty-seven. Another example is that of her grandmother Julia, who comes to mind when Francky speaks of "des gens qui refusent de sortir de leur lit et qu'on dit déprimés" (people who refuse to get out of bed and who are said to be depressed) (*FAS*, 68). As the writer-nurse revives figures from her family's past, she also reminds us of the proximity of individuals grappling with mental illness, suggesting that if we take a closer look, they are not distant from us and may even directly involve us.

Pineau pulls in the reader, refusing any distance between the *I* and *them* or *us*. Using the impersonal subject pronoun "*on*" ("we") in French, which refers to no one specifically but can mean one, people, you, they, he or she, or even I, the writer-nurse tells us, "Nul ne sait qui sera le prochain *on*" (No one knows who will be the next *one*), meaning the person who arrives at a psychiatric hospital. The writer-nurse provokes us: "*on* peut s'incarner en toi, ton père ou ta mère, ton enfant, ton amant, ta voisine, ta grand-mère chérie, ton mari, ton épouse, ton patron" (that one can be you, your father or your mother, your child, your lover, your neighbor, your beloved grandmother, your husband, your wife, your boss) (*FAS*, 13). Such a relational account of vulnerability might prevent us from perceiving it as weakness and incompatible with 'normality,' exploring instead its potential for proximity, understanding, and attention.

Pineau creates proximity not only through this uniting existential fragility but also by constituting a relational spatiality between hexagonal France and the French Caribbean. Although the writer-nurse worked for twenty years of her nursing career at the psychiatric hospital Saint-Claude in Guadeloupe, she centers the narrative of her experiences and encounters at a hospital in hexagonal France. This hexagonal perspective resists the constructing of madness as a naturalized historical and pathological condition specific to the Caribbean, which can be found, scholar Antonia Wimbush (2022) reminds us in her article about madness and Pineau's writing, in "the postcolonial discourse" that "reads madness as the enduring legacy of slavery and colonization" (170). This does not mean that instances of madness related to colonial and postcolonial violence are overlooked. Instead, by framing madness within the hexagonal context, Pineau preemptively counteracts its potential to be used as trope for othering and uncaring.

> Je viens d'une île, la Guadeloupe. Autrefois, enfant, je ramassais des coquillages sur la plage pour en faire des tableaux.... La plupart étaient émoussés, ébréchés, brisés.... Déjà, à l'époque, j'imaginais qu'ils avaient tous souffert de quelque chose.... Tels les coquillages jonchant les plages de la Guadeloupe, les personnes qui se trouvent à l'hôpital psychiatrique arrivent d'un long voyage. (*FAS*, 11–14)

> I come from an island named Guadeloupe. Long ago, as a child, I collected seashells on the beach to make pictures.... Most of them were dulled, chipped, broken.... Already then, I imagined that they had all been through some sort of suffering.... Like the

shells scattered across the beaches of Guadeloupe, people who arrive to the psychiatric hospital have been on a long journey.

Calling the analogy between the beached shells in Guadeloupe and patients an "'Atlantic' tactic," scholar Lorna Milne justly remarks on an expansive, "integrative" (to use her term) geographical and cultural imaginary that calls into question the postcolonial (post-1946) estrangement of the French Caribbean islands (2014, 217). For indeed, the imagery of vulnerability and fragility that takes shape in *Folie, aller simple* is one that encompasses humanity as a whole, and therefore stretches well beyond the French Caribbean context while also never deserting its shores.

Pineau retrieves from invisibilization the otherwise neglected voices of nurses, patients, and her own and the spaces they inhabit, including the psychiatric hospital and the French Caribbean. The writer-nurse concludes the narrative pondering on the words of an old psychiatric nurse she knew when she was practicing in Guadeloupe: according to him, "la folie des hommes était tout à fait naturelle. . . . Un jour, ils prennent conscience qu'ils sont condamnés à vivre là, sur cette maudite terre, au milieu des guerres et de la barbarie . . . [. . .] Ce monde est tellement invivable qu'ils renoncent et basculent dans un autre univers qui est celui de la folie, pour se sauver" (it was completely normal that people go mad. . . . One day, they realize that they are doomed to live here, on this damned earth, amid wars and brutality . . . [. . .] This world is so unbearable they give up and slip into madness to escape" (*FAS*, 202–203). The old nurse concluded, "Alors tu vois . . . , quand on soigne les fous, c'est nous-mêmes qu'on soigne, qu'on aide, qu'on réconforte. Tous ces grands malades sont des reflets de nous-mêmes dans le miroir" (So you see . . . , when we care for mad people, we care for ourselves too, we help and comfort ourselves. All these mad people are reflections of ourselves in the mirror) (*FAS*, 203–204). The mirror that they hold up to us reveals the devastating effect of uncaring, but also reflects the ways practices of care take shape and perhaps take hold.

Acknowledgments

I stumbled upon the concept of "care" somewhat unexpectedly. In the spring of 2019, while collaborating with my dissertation co-advisor, John Walsh, on a special issue on the theme of "Refugees between Aesthetics and Politics" (*Crossings: Journal of Migration and Culture*, 12: 1), we discussed inviting French scholar Fabienne Brugère to write the postface. Her work with Guillaume LeBlanc, *The End of Hospitality* (Flammarion, 2017), had been a significant source of inspiration for us, and we were thankful to have the opportunity to include her voice in that project. My collaboration with Fabienne Brugère extended further when I organized her virtual visit to discuss her work *Care Ethics: The Introduction of Care as a Political Category* (Peeters, 2019; originally published in French as *L'éthique du care*, PUF 2011), approximately a year after I started working at Georgetown University in the fall of 2020. Since then, the theories of care and the many voices that populate the field of care studies have profoundly influenced my thinking. I am thus forever grateful for that shared book obsession John and I had back in 2019.

I would now like to express my gratitude to the early readers of this book, in full or in part. I benefited greatly from their thoughtful feedback throughout the various stages of its writing. My most heartful thanks go to Leanne Doughty, Cae Joseph-Masséna, Susanna Lee, Anne O'Neil-Henry, and Lucy Swanson for your time and for asking the questions that needed be posed. My sincere thanks also go to Andrew Sobanet for being an incredible mentor and for his tireless and meticulous review of the drafts of my book proposal.

I am also grateful to the intellectual community I have found in the various seminars, colloquiums, and conferences that I have been able to attend and where I engaged in invigorating conversations about some of the texts and contexts that compose this study. I wish to note in particular, in chronological order, Antonia Wimbush and Jonathan Lewis, the organizers of the 2019 edition of the Society for Francophone Postcolonial Studies conference in London; Sylvia Grove and Amanda Vincent who joined me in conversation during the virtual roundtable "Practices of Care: Staying Connected to/through the Natural World" at the Twentieth and Twenty-First Century French and Francophone Studies International Colloquium in March 2021; Abigail Celis and Johanna Montlouis-Gabriel for organizing the panel "(Queer) Care—Decoloniality—Environmental Justice" at the *CFC Intersections* Inaugural Virtual Conference in March 2021, and my fellow participants—Abigail, Eric Disbro, Eirann Cohen, and Rachel Kirk—for their insightful contributions and intellectual engagement; Alexandre Gefen, Sandra Laugier, and Andrea Oberhuber who organized the "Caring Lit'/Pour une littérature du care" colloquium in Paris in October 2021; Dega Rutherford and Sara Mechkarini, organizers of the SFPS 2022 conference edition; and finally Gina Stamm and Cheryl Toman, organizers of the Women in French USA conference in March 2024.

My sincere thanks also go to the following people for inviting me to present my work, virtually or in person—I have deeply appreciated the encouragement, curiosity, and valuable feedback from my hosts and everyone in attendance at each event: Fabienne Brugère and Caroline Ibos, Paris 8 University; Patoimbasba Nikiema, University of Miami; and Dario Chimenti, Spencer Fricard, Casey Montgomery, and Hyunjin Kim, University of Pittsburgh.

My students at Georgetown University too have contributed greatly to my thinking about the multidisciplinarity and transregionality of the perspective of care. I wish to note in particular the students of my spring 2023 undergraduate seminar: Rose Becker, Nami Bolat, Caroline Ericsson, Meghan Gibbons, Juan González, Théa Jacquand, Isabel Janovsky, Sarah Khan, Katie Lefever, Jacqlyn Manu, Rebecca Ochan, Claire Smith, Brendan Teehan, and Chloe Vlases.

I would like to also extend my sincere thanks to Kim Guinta, former editorial director at Rutgers University Press, and Yolanda Martínez-San Miguel, Carter Mathes, and Kathleen López, editors of the series "Critical Caribbean Studies," for placing their trust in me from the outset of this project. I am also deeply grateful to Isabel Guzzardo Tamargo and Emma-li Downer at Rutgers University Press for their kindness and guidance.

In addition to the names already mentioned, I have been buoyed by the friendship and support of folks in both academic and personal circles. My heartfelt thanks go to my colleagues and friends at Georgetown University, especially those in my home department. I am also deeply grateful to the *Kwazman Vwa* community—Nathan Dize, Jocelyn Franklin, Corine Labridy, Erika Serrato, Lucy Swanson, and Charly Verstraet—for their unwavering solidarity and infectious good spirits. I give a special thank you also to John Walsh, who has consistently encouraged me to trust my instincts and has been a steadfast sounding board over the years. I would also like to acknowledge the friends and family who, often from afar, have shared in my excitement at every milestone and provided a constant breath of fresh air. My deepest thanks go especially to Yamodo and Wendy Akondjia, Emma Ben Hadj, Annie deSaussure, Quentin Fondecave, Sylvia Grove, Don Joseph, Charlotte Legendre, Thomas Lozano, Maonghe Mbaitjongue, Elian Moreau, Jessica Oublié and Vanessa Pénélope.

Portions of chapter 1 have been adapted from "Décryptage de l'exposition 'Le Modèle noir' au Musée d'Orsay, ou interroger l'évitement du passé colonial français par le biais de l'anonymat," *Francosphères* 10, no. 1 (2021). An edited version of the coda appeared under the title "Gisèle Pineau, or the Literary Voice of a Caregiver" in the special issue "The 21st-Century Social Novel in French," coedited by Loïc Bourdeau and Charly Verstraet, in *Nottingham French Studies* 63, no. 3 (2024): 253–263. I thank the publishers of both pieces for their kind permission to reprint that material here.

Most of all, I am indebted to my life partner, Leanne Doughty, for the beauty of our every day.

Finally, I dedicate this book to my triad, my pillars, my heart forever and always, Jules-Charles, Anne-Marie, and Amenophis Boum Make.

Notes

Introduction

1. Unless otherwise noted, all translations are my own.
2. *Merriam-Webster Thesaurus*, "care (n.)," accessed February 16, 2024. https://www.merriam-webster.com/thesaurus/care.
3. *Béké*, or white Creoles, is a term referring to the descendants of the original European, usually French, plantation owners and colonizers in the Antilles.
4. Overseas regions (commonly known as DOMs [Départements d'Outre-Mer], but administratively termed DROMs [Départements et Régions d'Outre-Mer] since the constitutional reform of 2003 transforming the territories into mono-departmental regions) are former colonies of France and have, since the law of departmentalization of 1946, the same administrative status as the thirteen regions in hexagonal France. The five DROMs are Guadeloupe, Martinique, Réunion, French Guiana, and Mayotte (since 2011). It is generally understood that French laws and regulations, like the civil code, tax laws, and penal code, apply to French overseas regions as they do in hexagonal France, but they can be adapted as needed according to the region's particular needs. Moreover, the local administrations of overseas regions cannot pass new laws.
5. On May 26, 1967, French police (CRS) brutally suppressed a workers' strike in Pointe-à-Pitre, Guadeloupe. After the killing of Jacques Nestor, a member of the pro-independence group GONG (Groupe d'Organisations Nationale de la Guadeloupe), tensions between the

protesters and the police quickly intensified. On May 26 and 27, a curfew was instituted, and a number of Guadeloupean protesters were killed by the police. Eighteen Guadeloupeans were arrested and put on trial in the French State Court of Security. The words quoted above were spoken by Aimé Césaire, then mayor and deputy for Martinique, during this trial (February 19 to March 1, 1968). For more on the May 1967 Massacre in Guadeloupe, see Dorlin and Rigouste (2023).

6. Lyannaj kont' Pwofitasyson (LKP) was formed from about fifty trade unions and social movements in Guadeloupe. LKP initiated in 2009 in the context of the historic mobilization of early 2009 in Guadeloupe against the high costs of living.

7. See the Facebook video by Jonathan Leury Agarat (2020). This collective of thirty-six organizations, associations, and unions was formed in 2018 following the Forum Social Zéro Chlordécone Zéro Pesticide, with the aim of sustaining and intensifying the battle against chlordecone pollution.

8. On the topic of mothering and in a Francophone North American context, see, for example, Bourdeau (2019).

9. This inquiry marks a departure from Tronto's definition of care because it broadens the scope for the application of care practices, a framework established in *Moral Boundaries*, where the scholar excludes literature ("creative activity," 105) from constituting a gesture of care, alongside activities such as "the pursuit of pleasure, . . . production, destruction . . . to play, to fulfill a desire, to market a new product." Tronto views caring as involving "taking the concerns and needs of the other as *the basis for action*" (105), suggesting that creating a work of art might have limited political impact in "real" life. Seeking to "elucidate" Tronto's logic, scholar Marjorie Deschênes argues for considering the historical position of artists and writers as "des 'puissants'" (the powerful) or "des 'privilégiés'" (the privileged): "les pratiques *caring* socialement déstabilisatrices ne peuvent provenir des artistes et écrivains, dominants parmi d'autres" (socially disruptive caring practices cannot originate from artists and writers, a privileged group among others) (2015, 221). However, Deschênes's interpretation of Tronto's skepticism

regarding the potential of literature to serve as a site for questioning, reorganizing, or reimagining practices of care seems rooted in a top-down homogenizing representation of writers and artists, which might be indicative of Tronto's original generalizing view.

10. Gefen's study offers a panorama of the latest works of fiction in French, exploring the perspective of restorative and/or therapeutic literature—that is, care narratives that may help redress the invisibility of microhistories as well as produce empathy, attention, and healing.

11. In her essay "Les ressources du récit chez Carol Gilligan et Paul Ricoeur: Peut-on penser une littérature *care*?" (2015), Deschênes proposes,

    Ce que j'appellerai au final la "littérature care," aussi bien du côté de la poétique des auteures que de celui de la critique littéraire, présenterait par ailleurs l'un ou l'autre de ces critères plus spécifiques: 1) les attitudes éthiques et temporelles qu'elle dépeint relèvent d'une égale attention à l'autre et à soi-même; 2) les personnages qu'elle figure rendent justice à la vulnérabilité et à la fragilité humaines; 3) un souci d'égalité entre les sexes ou les différentes identités y est présent, par exemple à travers une exigence de *mémoire* et de *promesse* (Ricœur, [1990] 2004) pour le groupe social "femmes" ou d'autres groupes historiquement minorisés; 4) elle critique le patriarcat et déboulonne les codes de genre. (222)

    (In the end, what I would call "caring literature," from the perspective of writers' poetics and literary criticism equally, would include one or the other specific criteria: 1) the ethical and temporal attitudes represented pay close attention to the self and the other; 2) characters do justice to human vulnerability and fragility; 3) preoccupation with equality between the sexes and other types of identities, expressed for example through the demand for *memory* and *promise* (Ricœur, [1990] 2004) with regard to "women" as a social group or other historically underrepresented groups; 4) a critique of patriarchy and the unraveling of gender norms.)

    Adding to the scholarly debates surrounding the classification of "caring literature," it is noteworthy to consider the insights offered by Canadian scholars Dominique Hétu and Maïté Snauwaert in their essay "Poétique et imaginaires du *care*" (2018). There, they caution against the potential risk of adopting a predominantly prescriptive and overly optimistic tone in defining the genre.

12. In the foreword, translated by Jeffrey Landon Allen, to the forthcoming volume *Graphic Narratives of Resistance: History, Politics, and Bandes Dessinées in French* (Edinburgh University Press), which I coedited with scholar Charly Verstraet.

Chapter 1   Curating Silences

1. See the section "La barque ouverte" (The open boat) in Glissant's *Poétique de la relation* (1990), 17–21.
2. See also the essay "Mama's Baby, Papa's Maybe: An American Grammar Book" (1987) by literary critic and Black feminist scholar Hortense Spillers, who describes the "cargo" of slave ships "packed like so many live sardines among the immovable objects" (70).
3. The British Library catalog mentions the wide outreach of the image used as a campaigning tool. A note includes that Thomas Clarkson explains in his *History of the Rise, Progress, and Accomplishment of the Abolition of the African Slave Trade* ([1808] 1968) that "the 'print seemed to make an instantaneous impression of horror upon all who saw it, and was therefore instrumental, in consequence of the wide circulation given it, in serving the cause of the injured Africans.'" The specific print was available from the British Library: https://web.archive.org/web/20200926063822/https://www.bl.uk/collection-items/diagram-of-the-brookes-slave-ship. See also "Brooks_(1781_ship)," Wikipedia, last modified November 11, 2024 15:37 (UTC), https://en.wikipedia.org/wiki/Brooks_(1781_ship).
4. The Parisian exhibition *Le modèle noir, de Géricault à Matisse* is in some respects a traveling exhibition. Originally developed by American scholar Denise Murrell, it was displayed at the Wallach Art Gallery at Columbia University from October 24, 2018, to February 10, 2019, under the name *Posing Modernity: The Black Model from Manet to Matisse to Today* (refer to the corresponding exhibition catalog; Murrell 2018). Another version of the exhibition I consider to a lesser extent in

this chapter was that curated by Jacques Martial, *Le Modèle noir: de Géricault à Picasso*. I regret missing the opportunity to attend the exhibition personally, but I did manage to acquire the educational dossier associated with the event, containing insightful curatorial commentary by Jacques Martial (Deriau-Reine and Louzon-Gamba 2019). It is worth noting also that the Guadeloupean rendition of the *Modèle noir* exhibition featured the same exhibition catalog as its Parisian counterpart.

5. See the work of scholars Renée Gosson, Anne-Claire Faucquez, and Androula Michael around arts and representations of colonial slavery in European museums.

6. Murrell's doctoral research completed in 2014 originates with the question "Who is the Black woman in Manet's *Olympia*?" because the discourse on the painting has centered almost exclusively on the nude woman, a prostitute lying on a bed and being brought flowers. Contrapuntally, Murrell describes her dissertation as an "attempt to provide a sustained art-historical treatment of the second figure, the prostitute's Black maid, posed by a model whose name, as recorded by Manet, was Laure." See Murrell's 2014 dissertation, "Seeing Laure: Race and Modernity from Manet's *Olympia* to Matisse, Bearden and Beyond."

7. Gilles Boëtsch and Pascal Blanchard (2016) argue that the concept of "race" originated in Europe; they associate the notion with Georges-Louis Leclerc de Buffon's theory in the eighteenth century, who "had [himself] borrowed Pierre-Louis Moreau de Maupertuis's idea of a 'white origin' of humanity in the Caucasus and a process of degeneration under the effects of climate, diet, and lifestyle" (49). They also take note of the erasure of the concept of "race" in the 1970–1980s although the concept was responsible for imposing a racial grid on the social order since the eighteenth century in France. For more on the invention of "race" and its resurgence, see their chapter in *Vers la guerre des identités?* (2016).

8. The introductory panel to the Parisian exhibition *Le modèle noir* reads as follows:

Les titres d'oeuvres sont l'héritage d'une histoire. Nombreux sont les titres anciens qui reflètent des marqueurs raciaux datés, tels que

'Nègre', 'mulâtre', 'câpresse', courants au XIXe et au début du XXe siècle, mais ne pouvant plus être d'usage de nos jours. La plupart ne disent rien de l'identité des modèles. Grâce aux recherches menées à l'occasion de cette exposition, nous sommes parvenus à identifier certains d'entre eux et proposons dans le cadre de cette exposition un nouveau titre mentionnant le nom du modèle lorsqu'il était connu.

Titles of artworks reflect a historical heritage. There are numerous old titles that convey dated racial markers such as "Negro," "mulatto," "câpresse" commonly used in nineteenth century and at the beginning of the twentieth century, but could not be used today. Most of those terms reveal nothing about the identity of models. Thanks to research led for the purpose of this exhibition, we have managed to identify some of the models and propose a new title including the name of the model when it was known.

9. For a description of the Rijksmuseum's program and its purported goal, see Siegal (2015).
10. Susan Waller (2017) goes further to describe the fate of models, in particular aging ones, "given their low wages and intermittent schedules." Waller cites in particular a letter to a friend by painter Paul Milliet where he recounts the arrival of models looking for work: "Not one [of the students] seemed aware that he was looking at a degraded human being who was overcome by misery; not one felt the least bit of pity" (35).
11. For the working class as subjects, consider, for example, the depiction of nanny figures in Jacques-Eugène Feyen's *Le baiser enfantin* (1865) or Édouard Manet's *Enfants aux Tuileries* (circa 1861–1862), or the presence of women domestics or companions in Georg Emanuel Opiz's *Le Palais Royal. Promeneurs du Palais Royal devant le Café de la Paix* (circa 1814–1831) or Édouard Manet's *Olympia* (1863).
12. The term "Negress" (or "Negro" in the masculine) used throughout this book is not used in a derogatory manner but rather inscribes the terminology in the context of racialization of slavery similar to the texts in which it appeared originally.
13. See the alphabetical directory of models who posed at the École des Beaux-Arts between 1901 and 1933 in the exhibition catalog of *Le modèle noir: de Géricault à Matisse* (Debray et al. 2019, 211–217).

14. References to Laure de Margerie and Édouard Papet's work can be found in their co-authored book *Facing the Other: Charles Cordier (1827–1905), Ethnographic Sculptor* (2004).
15. See in particular chapter 9 in Nelson (2010), "Vénus Africaine: Race, Beauty, and African-ness," 170–179.
16. It is important to note the historical thread linking care work and socioracial bias because during the BUMIDOM years from 1963 to 1982 Antillean women arriving from overseas departments were trained as cleaners and nannies. As a reminder, the BUMIDOM was, in the postwar era, a state agency spearheaded by Michel Debré to control emigration to hexagonal France, using the population to fill specific gaps in the workforce, usually unskilled and low-paid jobs in health care, transportation, and the domestic service sector. For more on the politicization and the long-lasting social effects of the BUMIDOM, see Germain (2010), and for more on the history of the state agency, see Pattieu (2016).
17. This quotation, taken from the transcript of a lecture delivered by Édouard Glissant on April 30, 1992, at the University of the West Indies, Mona, is also available in his 2008 article. See also *Mémoires des esclavages* (Glissant 2007).
18. *Merriam-Webster Dictionary*, "heir, noun," accessed February 16, 2024. https://www.merriam-webster.com/dictionary/heir.
19. Ouidah in southern Benin was a major slave-trading post from the seventeenth to the nineteenth centuries. It is before the captives would start walking to the ships that they would be made to circle the tree known as "l'Arbre de l'Oubli" or the "Tree of Forgetfulness." As they were becoming dizzy, the captives were believed to forget everything about their past so as to annihilate their rebellious thoughts. Today a statue marks the site where the tree stood, and the commemorative plaque reads as follows: "En ce lieu se trouvait l'arbre de l'oubli. Les esclaves mâles devaient tourner autour de lui neuf fois, les femmes sept fois. Ces tours étant accomplis, les esclaves étaient censés devenir amnésiques. Ils oubliaient complètement leur passé, leurs origines et leur identité culturelle pour devenir des êtres sans aucune volonté de réagir ou de se rebeller." (The tree of forgetfulness stood in this location.

The male captives had to go around it nine times, and seven times for the women captives. After having circled the tree, the enslaved would supposedly lose their memory. They would forget everything about their past, their origins and their cultural identity to turn into beings with no desire to take action or rebel.) For a photo of the plaque in situ, see Peace-on-earth.org, "L'arbre de l'oubli (the tree of forgetfulness)," Ouidah, Atlantique, Bénin, *Flickr*, October 13, 2016, https://www.flickr.com/photos/peace-on-earth_org/29996350500/in/photostream/.

Chapter 2   Voices of the BUMIDOM, or the Colonial Legacy of Care Work

1. Sylvain Pattieu provides a comprehensive investigation into the distribution of people who left with the BUMIDOM into sectors of the French industry. Charts clearly point to the gender distribution of these migrations, with the most represented sectors being construction and metal work for men and domestic work for women. See in particular charts 8 and 10 in Pattieu (2016).
2. See chart 3 in Pattieu's study (2016, 88). These numbers also include arrivals through family reunification.
3. De Jesus passed away in 1977 in São Paulo, so she never could have read or received any of Ega's work. Ega herself died in 1976, and *Lettres* was published in 1978.
4. The protests that took place in Fort-de-France in December 1959 reflected the increasing social tensions over economic disparity and the sharp decline in employment in part due to the declining sugar and rum industry, thirteen years after the departmentalization law. For more on the social and historical context in the overseas departments more generally, see the chapter "Les grandes migrations: Les Ultramarins" in Pap Ndiaye's *La condition Noire* (2008).
5. I insist on including this corpus, even if sometimes marginally, in order to highlight the array of texts that propagate knowledge of the stories, individual or collective, about the BUMIDOM.
6. In the graphic narrative *Péyi an nou* (2017), Jessica Oublié is depicted asking her close relations born and living in hexagonal France what

they know about their family history and their relationship to the overseas departments more generally. One of them (David) answers bluntly, "Je ne sais pas quelle était la vie de mes parents en Martinique, ni pourquoi ils sont venus en France . . . les parents antillais ne parlent pas beaucoup d'eux et de leur passé" (I don't know anything about my parents' life in Martinique, or why they came to France . . . Antillean parents don't talk much about themselves or their past) (14).

As this example shows, transmission of the difficult past has halted, or is at least rather limited between the generation born in the overseas departments and the next.

In the 2008 documentary *Jambé dlo* ("Crossing the sea" in Creole; directed by Emmanuelle Bidou and Fabienne Kanor), Kanor interviews the daughter of Gilbert Jean Marie Flore who left Martinique through the BUMIDOM with the prospect of working as a police chief. The young woman, Ophélia Jean-Marie Flore, concedes that she has very little interest in her father's life story:

C'est l'histoire de mon papa, c'est pas forcément la mienne. . . . C'est son histoire, il vit avec, on vit avec et on la connait mais ça s'arrête là. Moi je vais pas aller raconter toute l'histoire de mes ancêtres . . . je sais strictement rien que ce soit sur la Martinique, que ce soit sur ma grand-mère j'en sais pas plus que ça, sur mon grand-père non plus, sur mes arrière-grands-parents encore moins. J'ai pas besoin de savoir, je suis bien et voilà. Je me sens plus blanche, que basanée. . . . Je me sens blanche avant tout.

(It is my father's story, it is not necessarily mine. . . . It is his story, he lives with it, we live it, and we know it, but that's it. I'm not going to go around telling the history of my ancestors . . . I don't know anything about Martinique, I know nothing about my grandmother or my grandfather, and even less about my great-grandfathers. I don't need to know, I'm doing well, that's it. I feel more white than Black. . . . I'm white before anything else.)

7. Hillary Chute rightly differentiates between the graphic novel, which refers to works of fiction, and the graphic narrative, which includes modes other than fiction. As she describes it, "a graphic narrative is a

book-length work in the medium of comics" (2008, 453). This appears to be a crucial distinction, especially in the case of representations of historical realities, which, often concerning marginalized peoples, are occasionally misinterpreted as fiction. During her interview with the collective Kwazman Vwa in March 2021, Jessica Oublié recounts that the history of the BUMIDOM appeared to some as fictitious; she explained that "[*Péyi an nou*] était un roman graphique documentaire, et tous les personnages qui étaient à l'image étaient vrais" (*Péyi an nou* was a documentary *graphic novel*, and all characters in it were real). We see here that the translation of the term from the French may seem misleading because the designation "roman graphique" (graphic novel) largely applies to works of both fiction and nonfiction, compared with the appellation "récit graphique" (graphic narrative), for example.

8. See, for instance, Pascale Molinier's conceptual groundwork for understanding what care work is in *Le travail du care* (2013). See also "Paradoxes in the Invisibility of Care Work" by Sandra Laugier (2021), where the scholar articulates the stakes of an education in attention in the moment of sudden "visibility of the invisible" that the COVID-19 pandemic more forcibly brought out (65).

9. See in particular the piece by Molinier (2012). On the issue of depersonalization and care work, Molinier gives the example of the servants in Jean Cocteau's film *La Belle et la Bête* (Beauty and the Beast) where they are "reduced to candelabra arms or hands pouring jugs," representative of "a faceless availability which does not expect any reciprocity" (297). This depersonalization was perhaps even more evocatively depicted in the 1991 Disney adaptation.

10. In the preface to the 2021 edition of Ega's *Lettres*, Elsa Dorlin notes that from the opening of the center in 1965 more than 700 "ménagères" (maids) will be trained to learn "bonnes manières" (good manners) and "moeurs européennes" (European traditions) (13). All these terms convey some form of cultural dogmatism, both a way to model cultural norms for life in hexagonal France and an attempt to bridle expression of cultural particularities.

11. See Murdoch's entry on the BUMIDOM in *Postcolonial Realms of Memory* (2020). In Félix Germain's article "Jezebel and Victims: Antillean

Women in Postwar France, 1946–1974" (2010), he discusses in particular the unfulfilled expectations of Antillean women who left the French Antilles on the deceitful promise of social uplift: "[They intended] to stay away from this type of work [low-wage positions, especially live-in maids], which their mothers, grandmothers, and aunts had often performed for the islands' privileged mulattoes and *békés*" (483).

12. Ega signals the pervasiveness of the stereotyped representations largely applied to Black Antillean women that helped justify their disproportionate relegation to care work. For example, while at work, she overhears her female employer tell her husband, in response to his appreciation of Ega's diligence, that "Elles ont cela dans le sang, ces femmes-là!" (Those women have it in their blood!) (*LN*, 43). On another occasion, Ega is received by "Mme la Concierge" who proposes to hire her to clean a staircase without even knowing who she is, to Ega's surprise. The concierge tells her, "C'est par pour rien qu'on dit 'Travailler comme un Noir!' C'est pas pour vous vexer, mais c'est vrai!" (It is not without reason that we say, 'Work like a slave!' I don't mean to offend you, but it's true!) (*LN*, 86). Blackness (in relation to the Antilles) thus becomes commodified to form a labor pool of carers and to confine a predefined group of people to certain skills.

13. Taking into account the loss of value due to inflation, the purchasing power of 220 francs in 1962 (year during which Ega met Yolande) is the same as that of 342.63 euros in 2021. Keeping in mind that Yolande only receives 70 francs, her purchasing power is brought down to 109 euros (Source: Institut National de la Statistique et des Études Économiques, https://www.insee.fr/en/accueil).

14. Here, Ega makes a significant word choice with "maîtres" because she, at the same time, anticipates a criticism made by scholars and writers such as Alain Anselin (see, for instance, *L'émigration antillaise en France: La troisième île*, 1979) and Daniel Boukman (see, in particular, *Les Négriers*, 1978) who later compare the state-organized migration with the slave trade, calling it a "new slave trade."

15. Sylvain Pattieu notes that starting in the early 1970s the number of female domestic workers relatively decreased and instead the number of hospital workers increased (cleaning staff, nursing assistants, or

women training to become nurses). A graph report (*x* axis of 3,000) shows that, although the number of domestic workers among the population of female BUMIDOM migrants remained proportionally higher (over 600 in 1975 and slightly under 500 in 1979), the number of hospital service workers ("agents hospitaliers") climbed to over 200 in 1975 then drastically decreased by 1979 (close to zero). See chart 10 in Pattieu's study (2016, 96).

16. In *La poétique de l'espace* (The poetics of space; [1957] 2020), Gaston Bachelard gives primacy to the lived or inhabited space. The theorist focuses on the house as a protective place, one that provides safety and peaceful daydreaming. The space of the home thus appears as typified and provides an unproblematized at-homeness. See in particular chapter 1, "La maison: De la cave au grenier. Le sens de la hutte."

17. The term "*métropolitain*" literally refers to individuals born in hexagonal (i.e., Metropolitan) France, who have come to the overseas departments for personal or professional reasons. To be identified as "métro" denotes distinct geographic and cultural characteristics.

18. In the specific context of the BUMIDOM, the graphic narrative highlights an important distinction in the organization of migration flows from the overseas departments, pointing to the specific case of French Guiana, which in the 1960s remained largely underpopulated. Serge Mam-Lam-Fouck, a retired historian from the Université de Guyane, makes an appearance during a conversation between Oublié and Monique Milia-Marie-Luce, a historian from the Université des Antilles (pôle Martinique), to explain that following World War II the French government attempted to encourage migration to French Guiana through the Bipig (Bureau pour l'Installation des Personnes Immigrées en Guyane, or the Office for the Development of Emigration to Guiana) (28–30). Although a BUMIDOM office was created in 1969 that led to the departure of 2,685 Guyanese, its primary goal was to attract workers from the Hexagon or abroad.

19. Concerning the collection of information, Oublié explains, in the context of a workshop organized at the University of Pittsburgh in March 2019 on the theme "How to Tell the Hidden Histories of Migration in Graphic Narrative Form," that her investigation

methodology relied on a relational approach. Most of her investigative work was made possible through calls for testimonies, which led to interview phone calls or in-person meetings, combined with archival research.

20. For more on Simone Weil's conception of attention, see in particular "Réflexions sur le bon usage des études scolaires en vue de l'amour de Dieu" (Reflections on the right use of school studies with a view to the love of God) in *Attente de Dieu* (Waiting for God; 1966). The compilation of letters was written between January and May 1942. In *Attente de Dieu*, Weil's philosophical exploration of the concept provides a critical frame for thinking about the value and acquisition of attention in education but is not limited to it.

Chapter 3 Inhabiting the Land after Environmental Damage

1. In her analysis of paradisiacal tropes as part of a Caribbean canon, Lorna Burns (2008) comments on representations of the Caribbean as paradise since the early accounts of Columbus and all the way to what she calls "touristic myopia" (26) forming a set of misleading "exoticist imaginings" (33) that "disguis[e] the exploitation of its resources, but also the power relations that existed between coloniser and colonized" (26), as well as their lasting, unreckoned legacies well into the present.

2. In *Une écologie décoloniale* (2019), scholar Malcolm Ferdinand attributes three main principles to what he terms "l'habiter colonial" (or "colonial inhabitation"). The first concerns geography because inhabitation is "localisé au sein de la géographie de la Terre" (located within the geography of the Earth) as well as "géographiquement subordonnée à un autre lieu, à un autre espace" (geographically subordinate to another location, another space) in the sense of a ontological dependency on hexagonal France. The second concerns "l'exploitation des terres et de la nature" (the exploitation of the land and the nature of these islands) of colonized spaces, concomitant with a third principle, "l'altéricide" (othercide)—that is, "le refus de la possibilité d'habiter la Terre en présence d'un autre, d'une personne qui soit différente d'un moi par ses apparences ou ses croyances" (the refusal of the possibility of

inhabiting the Earth in the presence of an Other, a person who is different from a "self" in their appearance, their social affiliations, or their beliefs) (56–57, 28–29 in Anthony Paul Smith's translation, 2021).

3. RATP stands for Régie Autonome des Transports Parisiens. It is responsible for most of public transport in the Greater Paris area, including the Paris Métro, trams, buses, and regional express rail (RER) networks.

4. In the Caribbean, the word "mornes" designates hills and mountains of volcanic origins.

5. See, for example, Haitian painter Wilson Bigaud's *Paradis terrestre* (1953) or Salnave Philippe-Auguste's *Eve in the Garden of Eden* (1972).

6. These references constitute the necessary recognition of an area of study that brings into dialog violences against women and degradation of the nonhuman worlds. The term "ecofeminism" may be linked with the works of Françoise d'Eaubonne (notably *Le féminisme ou la mort* [1974] 2020) because she draws a parallel between the exploitation of the environment and the exploitation of women in the sense that these two forms of exploitation emanate from the same mode of inhabiting the world, one that is rooted in productivist capitalism and patriarchal oppression. One main problem, though, is that d'Eaubonne identifies the exploitation of women as pertaining to their reproductive power, pointing to the excess of births and therefore overpopulation, which she combines with the destruction of resources. But this hyperfocus on population control to deploy women's emancipation is reductionist for it fails to look at how societies, non-Western societies, and women in particular can operate differently elsewhere, and attempt to repair and maintain life against overaccumulation of capital and resources in the hands of a few—in short, against the conceptual impasse of the development/underdevelopment axis. Thinkers like Vandana Shiva and Maria Mies have, for that matter, shown the ways in which colonialism and its legacy has shaped destructive relations to the land and the oppression of women. They stress the need, especially for the dispossessed, to reclaim sustainable relationships with the land and refuse the passivity that has been imposed on women and nature.

7. To reflect the concrete particulars of the Caribbean, in particular the complex interrelation of multiple cultural identities, Glissant prefers the term "Détour," a strategy that is rather focused on the moment of entanglement, of coming into Relation and being transformed by it. See section 3 of the chapter "La dépossession" in *Le discours antillais* for more on "le Détour" ([1981] 1997, 48–57).
8. Tina Campt defines fugitivity as practices of refusal, complicating the act of flight as not just that of escape but also of defiance to racialized dispossession in quotidian practices of Black communities, in particular in the context of Black feminist futures. See *Listening to Images* (2017), especially chapter 1, "Quiet Soundings: The Grammar of Black Futurity" (15–45).
9. The story of Solitude was inspired by the life of Mulâtresse Solitude, a Maroon heroine in the fight against enslavement in Guadeloupe. Her life as recounted in the illustrated novel *Solitude la flamboyante* (2020) by Paula Anacaona (writer) and Claudia Amaral (illustrator) may be of interest to our understanding of *marronnage* as an in-the-world form of resistance. Solitude lives at Bellesource, a sugarcane plantation owned by the L'Arbresle family. Henriette, an older enslaved woman on the plantation, gradually inspires thoughts of resistance in Solitude's mind and prompts her to join the fight against enslavement. While still on the plantation, Solitude joins a network of resistance that forges documents, passes on secret correspondence, and steals provisions. "Donc j'étais Marronne" (So I was marooning), Solitude declares (90), locating *marronnage* in the disposition, the ability to disrupt and eventually dislodge normalized forms of oppression.
10. The essay translated by Patricia Paperman appears as part of a volume edited by Vanessa Nurock titled *Carol Gilligan et l'éthique du care* (2010). The collection of essays as a whole is an invitation to reflect on Gilligan's influential work on the liberation of caring and the defense of "different voices" against dominant patriarchal cultural norms. This particular essay is based on a conference paper given by Gilligan at the School for Advanced Studies in the Social Sciences (EHESS) on May 13, 2009, at the invitation of Patricia Paperman and Sandra Laugier on the occasion

of the release of the republication in French of *Une voix différente* (*In a Different Voice* [1982] 2008).

11. During a research trip to Hopewell in Virginia, Oublié describes her encounter with Gregory Wilson, an environmental history professor at the University of Akron. Wilson explained that Kepone was patented by Allied Chemical in 1952 to be used against banana pests in Latin America, Europe, and Africa, and was registered with federal agencies in 1957. In 1973, Life Science Products (LSP), in charge of Kepone production for Allied Chemical, began to dump its used water into the James River. By 1975, LSP employees were being hospitalized for Kepone poisoning, and water and fish samples were showing evidence of Kepone. On July 24, 1975, Virginia closed the factory after witnessing the health impact of Kepone on its factory workers. Following the Kepone scandal, the state of Virginia prohibited fishing in the James River for thirteen years to prevent further exposure to the toxin. The following year, in 1976, the U.S. Environmental Protection Agency (EPA) banned the use and manufacture of the chemical in the United States. Chlordecone was only banned globally by the Stockholm Convention on Persistent Organic Pollutants in 2009.

12. See the scientific information on soil and waterway contamination shown graphically and presented by Patrick Andrieux, hydropedologist and research engineer at the Institut National de la Recherche Agronomique (INRA) and Yves-Marie Cabidoche, then research director at INRA, who is resurrected in the shape of a genie (*TT*, 64–66). See also the literature about chlordecone poisoning in the French Caribbean in *Chronique d'un empoisonnement annoncé: Le scandale du chlordécone aux Antilles françaises 1972–2002* (2007) by Raphaël Confiant and Louis Boutrin.

13. In her study of gardens in Guadeloupe, *Corps, jardins, mémoires* (2000), Catherine Benoît makes mention of Félix Longin's 1848 *Voyage à la Guadeloupe* (2012, reprinted by the Société d'Histoire de La Guadeloupe) where Longin notes that the enslaved would receive a weekly ration of salt herring and cornmeal: "deux livres de morue et deux pots de farine pour les hommes, une livre et demie de morue et un pot et demi de farine pour les femmes (le pot de farine pèse environ deux

livres et demie)" (two pounds of herrings and two jars of cornmeal for the men, one pound and a half of herrings and one jar and a half of cornmeal for the women [the jar of cornmeal weighs about two pounds and a half]) (213).

14. See in particular chapter 3, "Jardins d'histoire" (95–128), in Benoît's study for her historical analysis of the functions of the *jardin créole*, one that produces food as well as has medicinal and ornamental value.

15. The Jafa program was established in 2009 by the Agence Régionale de Santé de Guadeloupe to reduce the exposure of local populations to chlordecone by pre-emptively assessing the levels of chlordecone in family gardens and helping to change habits of cultivation and consumption of animal and vegetable products if necessary. See the Jafa website at https://jafa.ireps.gp/.

16. *Online Etymology Dictionary*, "inhabit (v.)," accessed February 16, 2024, https://www.etymonline.com/search?q=inhabit.

17. As a side example, Oublié tells us about a common practice in viticulture in hexagonal France: the use of weed-killing products, pesticides, and fungicides against mildew or fungal infections. Attempting to draw an evocative parallel to the banana plantations in the French Caribbean (for an audience in hexagonal France), Oublié meets with Emmanuelle Piovesan who used to work as a viticulture consultant (115). Piovesan establishes a similar correlation between pesticide usage and illnesses such as cancers, respiratory diseases, and Parkinson's disease.

18. One recent example of governmental unresponsiveness occurred during the *Grand Débat* (the Great Debate), an initiative launched by President Macron across France in January 2019 to address social fractures in a series of local meetings and citizen assemblies amid the Gilets Jaunes protests. In a conversation with elected representatives from Guadeloupe and Martinique in February 2019 (recounted in the graphic narrative; *TT*, 96–97), Macron insisted that "Il ne faut pas aller jusqu'à dire que [le chlordécone] est cancérigène" (We cannot go so far as saying that chlordecone is carcinogenic). However, scientific research such as the Inserm (French National Institute of Health and Medical Research) study conducted in 2010 by Luc Multigner and

colleagues (2010) has shown that there is a significant increase in the risk of prostate cancer associated with chlordecone exposure.

19. The Kwazman Vwa (Crossing Paths) collective was founded by Nathan H. Dize, Corine Labridy, Erika Serrato, Jocelyn Sutton Franklin, Lucy Swanson, Charly Verstraet, and me. The collective aims to host digital conversations with emerging voices in the Caribbean world. Kwazman Vwa's inaugural event was hosted in February 2021 and featured an interview with Néhémy Pierre-Dahomey to discuss his novel *Rapatriés* (Seuil, 2017). Kwazman Vwa's homepage can be found at https://kwazmanvwa.com/. See the full interview (2021) with Jessica Oublié conducted by Charly Verstraet and myself at https://www.youtube.com/watch?v=EBDiodwCgio.

20. As a reminder, in *Le discours antillais* ([1981] 1997) Glissant suggests that "le rapport à la terre est d'autant plus menacé que la terre de la communauté est aliénée" ("the relationship with the land is even more threatened because the community is alienated from that land") (343; 1989, 105, translation by J. Michael Dash).

21. Lyannaj pou Dépolyé Matinik is a solidarity collective that was formed following the social forum "Zéro Chlordécone Zéro Pesticide" organized in April 2018 in Fort-de-France. The result of this forum was notably an outlining of fifty-two measures that highlight what is needed by local populations as a consequence of polluted living environments. The collective incorporates diverse organizations, unions, associations such as Agrikiltè pou ni tè, Assaupamar, and Santé et Environnement sans Dérogation (SESD), and members of the public, all coming together to participate in the effort to depollute Martinique.

22. In the documentary *Les derniers maîtres de la Martinique* (2009), Romain Bolzinger explains that "52% of all agricultural lands belong to less than 1% of the population." Such economic control is captured in *Tropiques toxiques* in the form of a diagram in which the *béké* monopoly over importing and exporting as well as local supermarkets is also made apparent: "Three large families share among each other 40% of the local supermarkets of the island" (*TT*, 174). In an economic and social context where the interests of the békés prevail, the extensive

use of chlordecone in banana plantations is linked solely to profitability with very little regard for human and nonhuman health or environmental pollution.

23. The term "caring deficit" appears in Tronto's study of the misallocation of caring responsibilities considering gender, race, class, and market forces in *Caring Democracy: Markets, Equality, and Justice* (2013). The scholar references the works of Katrin Bennhold (2011) and Sara Miller Llana (2006) where the notion is first used.

Chapter 4   Rebellious Care, or Deconstructing the Myth of the *Poto-mitan* Woman

1. Law XIII states, "We wish that if a slave husband has married a free woman, the children, both male and girls, will follow the condition of their mother and be free like her, in spite of the servitude of their father; and that if the father is free and the mother enslaved, the children will be slaves the same" (Louis XIV, 1685).
2. Ama Mazama, "Potomitan," in *Encyclopedia of African Religion* (Asante and Mazama 2009, 534–535). For an exploration of the extensive scholarship surrounding this archetype that upholds the values of strength, courage, and dedication in Caribbean girlhood and womanhood, refer to more comprehensive definitions of the *poto-mitan* image, such as N'Zengou-Tayo (1998), Mulot (2021), or Lamour (2021).
3. Scholar Michelle Rowley highlights an important difference between matrifocality and matriarchy by reminding us that "matrifocality [implies] a cultural and affective centrality of women within their kinship group. 'Matriarchy' . . . transcends notions of kinship and addresses not only the familial centrality of women, but also a centrality that extends to the ideological and institutional ordering of social organization." Rowley concludes, "This distinction suggests . . . that the Caribbean has never been a matriarchal region, by virtue of its matrifocality" (2002, 24).
4. In French, the substantive "bonne à tout faire" is formed from the adjective *bonne* (good) and the verbal phrase *tout faire* (do everything). In the text, then, following the repetition of the adjective "bon" to

describe the wife and the mother, the term "bonne à tout faire" (maid) appears to encapsulate all these identities.

5. In *Le discours antillais* (1997), Édouard Glissant presents the mother-father-child triad as a model that originated from the dominant *Béké* families in the French Caribbean yet was not popularized among enslaved populations, who were systematically denied the possibility of family formation. In a postslavery context, the nuclear family is imposed as a structuring societal force, but it clearly refutes the continuing legacy of slavery on interpersonal relationships as well as further "contredit [aux] tendances culturelles héritées de l'Afrique" (contradicts the cultural tendencies inherited from Africa) (168). These tendencies are, according to Glissant, "la forte amarre à la mère [avant] la période d'initiation" (the strong attachment to the mother before entering adulthood) and an expansive organization of the family ("la famille etendue," the extended family) to include only feminine figures: "soeurs aînées, tantes, marraines, grand-mères" (older sisters, aunts, godmothers, grandmothers) (166).

6. In many Caribbean and Latin American cultures, the rooster (*coq*) becomes a metaphor and symbol for masculinity, strength, and machismo. For more on the symbolism of the animal and cockfighting in particular, see Dundes and Bronner (2007).

7. In *La parole des femmes* (1979), Maryse Condé comments on the historical weight of the figurative castration of Black Caribbean men in the context of slavery (36), leading to the stereotype of sexually insatiable and irresponsible men—or "[l']étalon" (the stallion), to quote Glissant ([1981] 1997, 168)—in post-slavery societies as the reclamation of repressed masculinity. Importantly though, Condé reminds us that such stereotypical depictions of manhood should be contextualized within the broader framework of colonial and postcolonial history as well as the reality of socioeconomic relations in the Antilles.

8. In her analysis of Kanor's novel, Gladys Francis highlights Frida's murder-suicide as a "deconstruction of stereotypes and rigged discourses," in fact drawing inspiration from an interview with the author where Kanor herself supports this interpretation of the novel (2017, 105).

9. As a reminder, in their essay "Toward a Feminist Theory of Caring" (1990) Joan Tronto and Berenice Fisher propose that "caring can be viewed as a species of activity that includes everything that we do to maintain, continue, and repair 'our' world so that we can live in it as well as possible" (40).
10. In her analysis of *D'eaux douces*, Vété-Congolo interprets the title as the expression of an aspiration for more fresh waters to create a new relational ecosystem, free of salty ocean water, which symbolizes the legacy of the crossing of the Atlantic Ocean in the Middle Passage (2015, 118).
11. Compared to the other novel I study in this chapter, Octavia's text has received no scholarly attention to date. This might be explained by the fact that Octavia is primarily known as a playwright—her debut novel, *La fin de Mame Baby* was published in 2017.
12. Stéphanie Mulot (2009) has analyzed the dialectics between respectability and reputation alongside the gender binary. She revisits the scholarship on the meaning of respectability for women in Afro-Caribbean contexts, but Mulot also studies in greater detail male-specific attitudes of irresponsibility and unreliability that, she argues, must be understood as a consequence of sacralization of motherhood.
13. In *Introduction à la poétique du divers* (1996), Glissant, inspired by Gilles Deleuze and Félix Guattari's image of the rhizome, opposes the root-identity that "tue autour d'elle" (kills everything around it) (12). Rhizomatic thinking, which is inherently plural, "s'étend à la rencontre d'autres racines" (reach[es] out to different roots) (11). Translations by Célia Britton from *Introduction to a Poetics of Diversity* (2021).
14. Mulâtresse Solitude is a historical figure and national heroine of Guadeloupe, famous for her fight against slavery and French colonizers after having joined a community of Maroons in the late eighteenth century and early nineteenth century. According to André Schwarz-Bart's novel *La Mulâtresse Solitude* (1972), Solitude was hanged around 1802. Often depicted as pregnant, Solitude symbolizes to this day the strength and resilience of Caribbean women and mothers who fought for freedom and equality in the context of slavery. For more on Solitude, see also *Solitude la flamboyante* (2020), by Paula Anacaona and

illustrated by Claudia Amaral, a novel loosely inspired by the story of this historical figure in antislavery struggles of Afro-Caribbeans.

Coda

1. For more information regarding the "Caring lit/Pour une littérature du care" conference that took place in Paris in October 2021, see the introduction.
2. The *récit* opens with the sentence: "J'imagine immédiatement le corps de Sophie sur les rails du metro" (I immediately imagine Sophie's body on the metro train tracks) (9), indicating that Pineau has just learned about her death. The day at the hospital that the writer recounts takes place immediately after the passing of Sophie.
3. See the references to the theorists of care work such as Caroline Ibos, Sandra Laugier, Pascale Molinier, or Patricia Paperman, in chapter 3, "Voices of the BUMIDOM."
4. *Online Etymology Dictionary*, "delirium (n.)," accessed February 16, 2024, https://www.etymonline.com/search?q=delirium.

References

Abenon, Lucien, and Jacques Cauna. 1989. *Antilles 1789: La révolution aux caraïbes*. Nathan.

Agnant, Marie-Célie. 2002. *Le livre d'Emma*. Éditions du Remue-Ménage.

Anacaona, Paula, and Claudia Amaral. 2020. *Solitude la flamboyante*. Éditions Anacaona.

André, Jacques. 1987. *L'inceste focal dans la famille Noire antillaise: Crimes, conflits, structure*. Presses Universitaires de France.

Anselin, Alain. 1979. *L'émigration antillaise en France: La troisième île*. Anthropos Research.

Asante, Molefi Kete, and Ama Mazama, eds. 2009. *Encyclopedia of African Religion*. Sage.

Bachelard, Gaston. (1957) 2020. *La poétique de l'espace*. Presses Universitaires de France.

Baldwin, James. (1963) 2013. *The Fire Next Time*. Vintage Books.

Barbagallo, Camille, and Silvia Federici. 2012. "Introduction." In "Care Work and the Commons," edited by Camille Barbagallo and Silvia Federici. Special issue, *The Commoner* 15: 1–21. https://thecommoner.org/wp-content/uploads/2019/10/01-introduction.pdf.

Barthes, Roland. 1977. "From Work to Text." In *Image Music Text*, 155–164. Translated by Stephen Heath. Hill and Wang.

Benjamin, Walter. 2003. *The Arcades Project*. Translated by Howard Eiland and Kevin McLaughlin. Harvard University Press.

Bennhold, Katrin. 2011. "From Afar, Moneymaker and Mother." *New York Times*, March 7, 2011. https://www.nytimes.com/2011/03/08/world/europe/08iht-ffhelp08.html.

Benoît, Catherine. 2015. *Corps, jardins, mémoires: Anthropologie du corps et de l'espace à la Guadeloupe.* Les Éditions de la Maison des Science de l'Homme.

Bidou, Emmanuel, and Fabienne Kanor, dirs. 2007. *Jambé dlo: une histoire antillaise.* Mat Films/Telessonne/France 5. Vimeo, July 21, 2012. https://vimeo.com/46167329.

Bindman, David. 2017. "The Black Figure in the European Imaginary: An Introduction." In *The Black Figure in the European Imaginary*, edited by Adrienne L. Childs and Susan H. Libby, 11–15. D. Giles Limited.

Boëtsch, Gilles, and Pascal Blanchard. 2016. "Le retour de la 'race' dans les discours publics et scientifiques." In *Vers la guerre des identités? De la fracture coloniale à la révolution ultranationale*, edited by Pascal Blanchard, Nicholas Bancel, and Dominic Thomas, 47–58. La Découverte.

Bolzinger, Romain, dir. 2009. *Les derniers maîtres de la Martinique.* Canal+.

Boni, Tanella. 2018. *Habiter.* Museo.

Boukman, Daniel. 1978. *Les Négriers.* L'Harmattan.

Bourdeau, Loïc, ed. 2019. *Horrible Mothers: Representations across Francophone North America.* University of Nebraska Press.

Bourdeau, Loïc, Natalie Edwards, and Steven Wilson. 2020. "The Care (Re)Turn in French and Francophone Studies Introduction: Caring Relations." *Australian Journal of French Studies* 57 (3): 287–292. https://doi.org/10.3828/ajfs.2020.25.

Boutrin, Louis, and Raphaël Confiant. 2007. *Chronique d'un empoisonnement annoncé: Le scandale du chlordécone aux Antilles Françaises 1972–2002.* Éditions l'Harmattan.

Brugère, Fabienne. 2008. *Le sexe de la sollicitude.* Seuil.

———. (2011) 2021. *L'éthique du care.* Que Sais-Je.

Burns, Lorna. 2008. "Landscape and Genre in the Caribbean Canon: Creolizing the Poetics of Place and Paradise." *Journal of West Indian Literature* 17 (1): 20–41. http://www.jstor.org/stable/23019970.

Calhoun, Doyle. 2021. "A Fugue for the Middle Passage? Suicidal Resistance Takes Flight in Fabienne Kanor's *Humus* (2006)." *The French Review* 95 (2): 127–144. https://doi.org/10.1353/tfr.2021.0267.

Campt, Tina M. 2017. *Listening to Images.* Duke University Press.

The Care Collective. 2020. *The Care Manifesto: The Politics of Interdependence*. Verso.

Célestine, Audrey. 2018. *La fabrique des identités*. Karthala.

Chabanne, Vivien. 2020. "Faut-il renommer la Négresse aux pivoines?" Dossier pédagogique, January 8, 2020. Musée Fabre à Montpelier. https://pedagogie.ac-montpellier.fr/faut-il-renommer-la-negresse-aux-pivoines.

Chancy, Myriam J. A. 1997. *Framing Silence: Revolutionary Novels by Haitian Women*. Rutgers University Press.

Charon, Rita. 2001. "The Patient-Physician Relationship. Narrative Medicine: A Model for Empathy, Reflection, Profession, and Trust." *JAMA* 286 (15): 1897–1902. https://doi.org/10.1001/jama.286.15.1897.

Childs, Adrienne L., and Susan H. Libby, eds. 2017. *The Black Figure in the European Imaginary*. D. Giles Limited.

Chute, Hillary. 2008. "Comics as Literature? Reading Graphic Narrative." *PMLA* 123 (2): 452–465. http://www.jstor.org/stable/25501865.

Clarkson, Thomas. (1808) 1968. *The History of the Rise, Progress and Accomplishment of the Abolition of the African Slave-Trade by the British Parliament*. F. Cass and Co.

Condé, Maryse. 1979. *La parole des femmes: Essai sur des romancières des Antilles de langue française*. L'Harmattan.

Condon, Stéphanie, and Celia Britton. 2020. "Individual Strategies and State Strategies: The Shaping of French Caribbean Emigration by Gender Relations." *Clio: Women, Gender, History*, no. 51): 119–142. https://www.jstor.org/stable/27076667.

Curier, Charlise. 2019. *Mon aventure avec le BUMIDOM*. Éditions Nestor.

Curmer, Léon-Henri, ed, 1840–1842. *Les français peints par eux-mêmes: Encyclopédie morale du dix-neuvième siècle*. 9 vols. Louis Curmer Éditeur.

Curtius, Anny Dominique. 2010. "Utopies du BUMIDOM: Construire l'avenir dans un 'là-bas' postcontact." *French Forum* 35 (2–3): 135–155. https://doi.org/10.1353/frf.2010.0012.

D'Eaubonne, Françoise. (1974) 2020. *Le féminisme ou la mort*. Clandestin.

Debray, Cécile, Stéphane Guégan, Denise Murrell, and Isolde Pludermacher. 2019. *Le modèle noir, de Géricault à Matisse*. Musée D'Orsay/Flammarion.

Degras, Priska. 2011. *L'obsession du nom dans le roman des Amériques*. Karthala.

De Jesus, Carolina Maria. (1960) 2003. *Child of the Dark*. Signet Classic.

DeLoughrey, Elizabeth, Renée K. Gosson, and George B. Handley, eds. 2005. *Caribbean Literature and the Environment: Between Nature and Culture*. University of Virginia Press.

De Margerie, Laure, and Édouard Papet. 2004. *Facing the Other: Charles Cordier (1827–1905) Ethnographic Sculptor*. Harry N. Abrams.

Deriau-Reine, Sonia, and Aurélien Louzon-Gamba. 2019. *Dossier Pédagogique*. https://web.archive.org/web/20201108111235/https://pedagogie.ac-guadeloupe.fr/sites/default/files/File/ccruz/dossier_peda_le_modele_noir.pdf.

Derrida, Jacques. 1995. *Mal d'archive*. Éditions Galilée.

Deschênes, Marjorie. 2015. "Les ressources du récit chez Carol Gilligan et Paul Ricœur: Peut-on penser une littérature care?" In *Le care: Éthique féministe actuelle*, edited by Sophie Bourgault and Julie Perreault, 181–219. Éditions du Remue-Ménage.

Diallo, Rokhaya, and Grace Ly. 2020. "#56—Antilles Empoisonnées: Le Scandale Du Chlordécone." YouTube, November 24, 2020. https://www.youtube.com/watch?v=3T6v011Sg9o.

Diawara, Manthia, dir. 2010. *Édouard Glissant: One World in Relation*. Maumaus/Lumiar Cité.

D'Orlando, Natacha, Cécile Chapon, and Marine Cellier. 2020. "L'Alléluia des femmes-jardins: Perspectives écoféministes dans quelques œuvres de Jamaica Kincaid et Gisèle Pineau." *MaLiCE* 22. https://hal.science/hal-04044857.

D'Orlando, Natacha, and Tina Harpin. 2021. "Jardins Créoles, diasporas et sorcières: Lectures de l'écoféminisme caribéen." *Littérature* 201 (1): 82–98. https://doi.org/10.3917/litt.201.0082.

Dorlin, Elsa. 2022. *Self Defense: A Philosophy of Violence*. Translated by Kieran Aarons. Verso.

Dorlin, Elsa, and Mathieu Rigouste. 2023. *Guadeloupe, Mai 67: massacrer et laisser mourir*. Libertalia.

Dufoix, Stéphane. 2023. *Décolonial*. Anamosa.

Dundes, Alan, and Simon J. Bronner. 2007. "Gallus as Phallus: A Psychoanalytic Cross-Cultural Consideration of the Cockfight as Fowl

Play." In *Meaning of Folklore: The Analytical Essays of Alan Dundes*, edited by Simon J. Bronner, 285–316. University Press of Colorado. https://doi.org/10.2307/j.ctt4cgrzn.20.

Ega, Françoise. (1978) 2021. *Lettres à une Noire: Récit antillais.* Lux.

Fanon, Frantz. 1966. *The Wretched of the Earth.* Translated by Constance Farrington. Grove Press.

Federici, Silvia. 1975. *Wages against Housework.* Power of Women Collective/Falling Wall Press.

Ferdinand, Malcolm. 2019. *Une écologie décoloniale: Penser l'écologie depuis le monde Caribéen.* Seuil.

———. 2022. *Decolonial Ecology: Thinking from the Caribbean World.* Translated by Anthony Paul Smith. Polity Press.

Foucault, Michel. 2013. *History of Madness.* Routledge.

Francis, Gladys M. 2016. "Entretien avec Fabienne Kanor, 'L'Ante-Llaise par Excellence': sexualité, corporalité, diaspora et créolité." *French Forum* 41 (3): 273–288. https://doi.org/10.1353/frf.2016.0035.

———. 2017. *Odious Caribbean Women and the Palpable Aesthetics of Transgression.* Lexington Books.

Fuentes, Marisa J. 2016. *Dispossessed Lives: Enslaved Women, Violence, and the Archive.* University of Pennsylvania Press.

Gefen, Alexandre. 2018. *Réparer le monde: La littérature française face au XXIe siècle.* Éditions Corti.

Germain, Félix. 2010. "Jezebels and Victims: Antillean Women in Postwar France, 1946–1974." *French Historical Studies* 33 (3): 475–495. https://doi.org/10.1215/00161071-2010-006.

Gilligan, Carol. 1982. *In a Different Voice: Psychological Theory and Women's Development.* Harvard University Press.

———. 2006. "Une voix différente." In *Le souci des autres: Éthique et politique du care,* edited by Patricia Paperman and Sandra Laugier, Éditions de l'École des Hautes Études en Sciences Sociales (EHESS).

———. 2008. *Une voix différente: Pour une éthique du care.* Rev. ed. Translated by Annick Kwiatek. Flammarion. First published in English in 1982.

———. 2010. "Une voix différente: Un regard prospectif à partir du passé." In *Carol Gilligan et l'éthique du care,* edited by Vanessa Nurock, 19–38. Presses Universitaires de France.

Glenn, Evelyn Nakano. 2012. *Forced to Care: Coercion and Caregiving in America*. Harvard University Press.

———. 2000. "Creating a Caring Society." *Contemporary Sociology* 29 (1): 84–94. https://doi.org/10.2307/2654934.

Glissant, Édouard. 1964. *Le quatrième siècle*. Gallimard.

———. (1981) 1997. *Le discours antillais*. 1981. Gallimard.

———. 1989. *Caribbean Discourse: Selected Essays*. Translated by J. Michael Dash. University Press of Virginia.

———. 1990. *Poétique de la relation*. Gallimard.

———. 1996. *Introduction à la poétique du divers*. Gallimard.

———. 1997. *Poetics of Relation*. Translated by Betsy Wing. University of Michigan Press.

———. 2001. *The Fourth Century*. Translated by Betsy King. University of Nebraska Press.

———. 2007. *Mémoires des esclavages*. Gallimard.

———. 2008. "Creolization in the Making of the Americas." *Caribbean Quarterly* 54 (1/2): 81–89. https://www.jstor.org/stable/40655153.

———. 2020. *Introduction to a Poetics of Diversity*. Translated by Celia Britton. Liverpool University Press.

Glover, Kaiama L. 2021. *A Regarded Self: Caribbean Womanhood and the Ethics of Disorderly Being*. Duke University Press.

Griffin, Susan. 1978. *Woman and Nature: The Roaring Inside Her*. Harper & Row.

Gyssels, Kathleen. 2008. "Le 'poteau mitan,' du péristyle vaudou à la famille matrifocale." *Potomitan*, July 12, 2008. https://www.potomitan.info/penteng/potomitan.php.

Hache, Emilie, ed, 2016. *Reclaim: Recueil de textes écoféministes*. Cambourakis.

Haraway, Donna. 2015. "Anthropocene, Capitalocene, Plantationocene, Chthulucene: Making Kin." *Environmental Humanities* 6 (1): 159–165. https://doi.org/10.1215/22011919-3615934.

Harpin, Tina. 2017."'Adieu Madras, Adieu Foulard' ? Retour au pays et réflexion sur le genre dans trois œuvres d'écrivaines antillaises: *L'autre qui danse* de Suzanne Dracius (1989), *Lucy* de Jamaica Kincaid (1990) et *Combien de solitudes* de Véronique Kanor (2013)." In *Écrire et penser le genre en contextes postcoloniaux*, edited by Anne Castaing and Élodie Gaden, 91–112. Peter Lang.

Hartman, Saidiya. 2008. "Venus in Two Acts." *Small Axe: A Caribbean Journal of Criticism* 26 (2): 1–14. https://muse.jhu.edu/article/241115.

Herbeck, Jason. 2013. "Entretien Avec Fabienne Kanor." *The French Review* 86 (5): 964–976, https://www.jstor.org/stable/23511427.

Hirsch, Marianne. 2004. "Editor's Column: Collateral Damage." *PMLA* 119 (5): 1209–1215. https://www.jstor.org/stable/25486117.

Hirschman, Albert O. 1970. *Exit, Voice, and Loyalty: Responses to Decline in Firms, Organizations, and States*. Harvard University Press.

Hochschild, Arlie. 2014. "Global Care Chains and Emotional Surplus Value." In *Justice, Politics, and the Family*, edited by Daniel Engster and Tamara Metz, 249–261. Routledge.

hooks, bell. 1990. "Homeplace: a site of resistance." In *Yearning: Race, Gender, and Cultural Politics*, 41–49. Routledge.

Ibos, Caroline, Aurélie Damamme, Pascale Molinier, and Patricia Paperman. 2019. *Vers une société du care: Une politique de l'attention*. Le Cavalier Bleu.

Jean-Charles, Régine Michelle. 2021. "Getting around the Poto Mitan: Reconstructing Haitian Womanhood in the Classroom." In *Teaching Haiti: Strategies for Creating New Narratives*, edited by Cécile Accilien, and Valérie K. Orlando, 15–33. University Press of Florida. https://www.jstor.org/stable/j.ctv1t2mz45.5.

———. 2022. *Looking for Other Worlds: Black Feminism and Haitian Fiction*. University of Virginia Press.

Jean-François, Emmanuel Bruno. 2017. "Espace océanique, parole archipélique et polyphonie mémorielle dans *Humus* de Fabienne Kanor." *Women in French Studies* 25: 77–92. https://doi.org/10.1353/wfs.2017.0006.

Kanor, Fabienne. 2004. *D'eaux douces: roman*. Gallimard.

———. 2006. *Humus*. Gallimard.

———. 2020. *Humus*. Translated by Lynn E. Palermo. University of Virginia Press.

Kincaid, Jamaica. 2020. "The Disturbances of the Garden." *New Yorker*, August 31, 2020. https://www.newyorker.com/magazine/2020/09/07/the-disturbances-of-the-garden.

Kwazman Vwa. 2021. "Kwazman Vwa Presents an Interview with Jessica Oublié, Author of *Tropiques Toxiques*." YouTube, June 8, 2021. https://www.youtube.com/watch?v=EBDiodwCgio.

Lamour, Sabine. 2021. "Between Intersectionality and Coloniality: Rereading the Figure of the Poto-Mitan Woman in Haiti." *Women, Gender, and Families of Color* 9 (2): 136–151. https://doi.org/10.5406/23260947.9.2.02.

Larose, Véronique. 2007. "Fabienne KANOR—Identité d'une féminité Noire: Son roman *D'eaux douces* (2024)." *Potomitan: Pawol Kreyol*, 2007. https://www.potomitan.info/atelier/pawol/kanor.php.

Larrier, Renée. 1998. "A Roving 'I': 'Errance' and Identity in Maryse Condé's *Traversée de la Mangrove*." *L'Esprit Créateur* 38 (3): 84–94. https://www.jstor.org/stable/26288167.

Laugier, Sandra. 2015. "Voice as Form of Life and Life Form." Special issue, *Nordic Wittgenstein Review* 4: 63–82. https://doi.org/10.15845/nwr.v4i0.3364.

———. 2021. "Paradoxes in the Invisibility of Care Work." *Philosophical Topics* 49 (1): 61–79. https://doi.org/10.5840/philtopics20214915.

Lebastard, Léa. 2024. "Accès à l'eau: 'L'État est responsable de la mise en danger des Guadeloupéens.'" *Politis*, March 21, 2024. https://www.politis.fr/articles/2024/03/guadeloupe-acces-a-leau-letat-est-responsable-de-la-mise-en-danger-des-guadeloupeens.

Lefaucheur, Nadine. 2018. "Situations monoparentales à la Martinique et idéal sacrificiel du potomitan." *Revue des Politiques Sociales et Familiales* 127 (1): 23–35. https://doi.org/10.3406/caf.2018.3283.

Leury Agarat, Jonathan. 2020. "Doubout pou lavi san chlordecone san pies pestisid!" *Facebook*, November 5, 2020. https://www.facebook.com/jonathanleuryagarat/videos/1484614998402646/.

Lionnet, Françoise. 2021. *Le su et l'incertain: Cosmopolitiques créoles de l'Océan Indien*. L'Atelier d'écriture.

Llana, Sara Miller. 2006. "Global Stopgap for US Nurse Deficit." *Christian Science Monitor*, March 6, 2006. https://www.csmonitor.com/2006/0306/p02s01-usec.html.

Loichot, Valérie, and Gisèle Pineau. 2007. "'Devoured by Writing': An Interview with Gisèle Pineau." *Callaloo* 30 (1): 328–337. https://doi.org/10.1353/cal.2007.0152.

Longin, Félix. 2012. *Voyage à la Guadeloupe (1816–1822)*. Société d'Histoire de La Guadeloupe.

Lorde, Audre. (1984) 2007. "The Transformation of Silence into Language and Action." In *Sister Outsider: Essays and Speeches*, 40–44. Crossing Press.

Louis XIV. 1685. *Le Code Noir ou recueil des règlements rendus jusqu'à présent* (Paris: Prault, 1767). Translated by John Garrigus. Société d'Histoire de la Guadeloupe, 1980. https://s3.wp.wsu.edu/uploads/sites/1205/2016/02/code-noir.pdf.

Maestrati, Antoine-Léonard, dir. 2007. *L'avenir est ailleurs*. Cinéma Public Films.

Mangangu, Bona. 2016. *Joseph Le Maure*. Createspace Independent Publishing Platform.

Martin, Laurent. 2020. "'Le modèle noir, de Géricault à Matisse': Un modèle d'exposition." *Sociétés et Représentations* 1 (49): 235–238. https://doi.org/10.3917/sr.049.0235.

Maximin, Daniel. 2006. *Les fruits du cyclone: Une géopoétique de la Caraïbe*. Seuil.

Memmi, Dominique. 2016. "Aides à domicile et domination rapprochée." *La Vie des Idées*, May 4, 2016. https://laviedesidees.fr/Aides-a-domicile-et-domination-rapprochee.

Merchant, Carolyn. 1980. *The Death of Nature: Women, Ecology, and the Scientific Revolution*. HarperOne.

Mies, Maria, and Vandana Shiva. 1993. *Ecofeminism*. Zed Books.

Mignolo, Walter, and Catherine E. Walsh. 2018. *On Decoloniality: Concepts, Analytics, Praxis*. Duke University Press.

Miller, Ann. 2007. *Reading Bande Dessinée: Critical Approaches to French-Language Comic Strip*. Intellect Books.

Milne, Lorna. 2014. "Working, Writing and the Antillean Postcolony: Patrick Chamoiseau and Gisèle Pineau." *Paragraph* 37 (2): 205–220. https://doi.org/10.3366/para.2014.0122.

Mitchell, Robin. 2020. *Vénus Noire: Black Women and Colonial Fantasies in Nineteenth-Century France*. University of Georgia Press.

Mohammed, Patricia, ed. 2002. *Gendered Realities: Essays in Caribbean Feminist Thought*. Mona, Jamaica: Centre for Gender and Development Studies.

Molinier, Pascale. 2006. "Le care à l'épreuve du travail." In *Le souci des autres: Éthique et politique du care*, edited by Patricia Paperman and Sandra Laugier, 339–357. Éditions de l'École des Hautes Études en Sciences Sociales (EHESS).

———. 2012. "Of Feminists and Their Cleaning Ladies." In "Care Work and the Commons," edited by Silvia Federici and Camille Barbagallo. Special issue, *The Commoner* 15: 286–305. https://thecommoner.org/wp-content/uploads/2019/10/13-molinier.pdf.

———. 2013. *Le travail du care*. La Dispute.

Molinier, Pascale, Sandra Laugier, and Jules Falquet, eds. 2015. *Genre et environnement: Nouvelles menaces, nouvelles analyses au Nord et au Sud*. L'Harmattan.

Molinier, Pascale, Sandra Laugier, and Patricia Paperman, eds. (2009) 2021. *Qu'est-ce que le care? Souci des autres, sensibilité, responsabilité*. Éditions Payot.

Morgan, Jennifer L. 2021. *Reckoning with Slavery: Gender, Kinship, and Capitalism in the Early Black Atlantic*. Duke University Press.

Mulot, Stéphanie. 2000. "'Je suis la mère, je suis le père!': L'énigme matrifocale. Relations familiales et rapports de sexe en Guadeloupe." PhD diss., Ecole des Hautes Etudes en Sciences Sociales. https://theses.hal.science/tel-00266923.

———. 2009. "Redevenir un homme en contexte antillais post-esclavagiste et matrifocal." *Autrepart* 49 (1): 117–135. https://doi.org/10.3917/autr.049.0117.

———. 2021. "Peut-on être guadeloupéenne, *potomitan* et féministe?" *Recherches Féministes* 34 (2): 123–148. https://doi.org/10.7202/1092234ar.

Multigner, Luc, Jean Rodrigue Ndong, Arnaud Giusti, Marc Romana, Helene Delacroix-Maillard, Sylvaine Cordier, Bernard Jégou, Jean Pierre Thome, and Pascal Blanchet. 2010. "Chlordecone Exposure and Risk of Prostate Cancer." *Journal of Clinical Oncology* 28 (21): 3457–3462. https://doi.org/10.1200/jco.2009.27.2153.

Murdoch, Adlai H. 2020. "BUMIDOM." In *Postcolonial Realms of Memory: Sites and Symbols in Modern France*, edited by Etienne Achille, Charles Forsdick, and Lydie Moudileno, 244–254. Liverpool University Press.

———, ed. 2021. *The Struggle of Non-Sovereign Caribbean Territories.* Rutgers University Press.

Murray-Román, Jeannine. 2022. "Care Webs and the Creole Garden in Manthia Diawara's *Édouard Glissant: One World in Relation.*" *French Screen Studies* 22 (1): 77–90. https://doi.org/10.1080/26438941.2021.2003555.

Murrell, Denise M. 2014. "Seeing Laure: Race and Modernity from Manet's *Olympia* to Matisse, Bearden and Beyond." PhD diss., Columbia University. https://academiccommons.columbia.edu/doi/10.7916/D8MK69VP.

———. 2018. *Posing Modernity: The Black Model from Manet and Matisse to Today.* Yale University Press.

Ndiaye, Pap. 2008. *La condition Noire: Essai sur une minorité française.* Calmann-Lévy.

Nelson, Charmaine A. 2010. *Representing the Black Female Subject in Western Art.* Routledge.

Ni Cheallaigh, Gillian, Laura Jackson, and Siobhán McIlvanney, eds. 2014. *Quand La Folie Parle: The Dialectic Effect of Madness in French Literature since the Nineteenth Century.* Cambridge Scholars.

N'Zengou-Tayo, Marie-José. 1998. "'Fanm Se Poto Mitan: Haitian Woman, the Pillar of Society." *Feminist Review* 59 (1): 118–142. https://doi.org/10.1080/014177898339497.

Oberhuber, Andrea, and Alexandre Gefen. 2022. "Souci d'autrui, soin, écriture." In "Pour une littérature du care," edited by Alexandre Gefen, Andrea Oberhuber, and Antoine Poisson. Special issue, *Fabula, Colloques.* https://doi.org/10.58282/colloques.8305.

Octavia, Gaël. 2020. *La bonne histoire de Madeleine Démétrius.* Gallimard.

Oublié, Jessica. Forthcoming. "Foreword." Translated by Jeffrey Landon Allen. In *Graphic Narratives of Resistance: History, Politics, and Bandes Dessinées in French*, edited by Jennifer Boum Make and Charly Verstraet. Edinburgh University Press.

Oublié, Jessica, Nicola Gobbi, Katherine Avraam, and Vinciane Lebrun. 2020. *Tropiques toxiques: Le scandale du chlordécone.* Steinkis.

Oublié, Jessica, and Marie-Ange Rousseau. 2017. *Péyi an Nou.* Steinkis.

Owens, Emily. 2016. "Enslaved Women, Violence, and the Archive: An Interview with Marisa Fuentes." *African American Intellectual History*

Society: Black Perspectives, October 4, 2016. https://www.aaihs.org/enslaved-women-violence-and-the-archive-an-interview-with-marisa-fuentes/.

Paperman, Patricia, and Sandra Laugier, eds. 2006. *Le souci des autres: Éthique et politique du care*. Éditions de l'École des Hautes Études en Sciences Sociales (EHESS).

Pattieu, Sylvain. 2016. "Un traitement spécifique des migrations d'Outre-Mer: Le BUMIDOM (1963–1982) et ses ambiguïtés." *Politix* 116 (4): 81–113. https://doi.org/10.3917/pox.116.0081.

———. 2021. "BUMIDOM 1963–82: Organizing Overseas Migrations to the Metropole, Actions and Contradictions." In *The Black Populations of France: Histories from Metropole to Colony*, edited by Sylvain Pattieu, Emmanuelle Sibeud, and Tyler Stovall, 123–138. University of Nebraska Press.

Persson, Ann-Sofie. 2017. "'Il faut souffrir pour être belle': Constructions de la féminité dans *D'eaux douces* de Fabienne Kanor." *Women in French Studies* 25 (1): 68–76. https://doi.org/10.1353/wfs.2017.0005.

Pierre-Dahomey, Néhémy. 2017. *Rapatriés*. Seuil.

Pineau, Gisèle. (1996) 2000. *L'exil selon Julia*. Le Livre de Poche.

———. 2008. *Morne Câpresse*. Folio.

———. 2010. *Folie, aller simple: Journée ordinaire d'une infirmière*. Philippe Rey.

———. 2013. *Mes quatre femmes*. 2007. Philippe Rey.

Rancière, Jacques. (1992) 2014. *Les noms de l'histoire: Essai de poétique du savoir*. Seuil.

Renaud, Leighan. 2020. "Beyond the Nuclear: The Caribbean Family." *History Workshop*, August 12, 2020. https://www.historyworkshop.org.uk/Black-history/beyond-the-nuclear-the-caribbean-family/.

Ricœur, Paul. (1990) 2004. *Soi-même comme un autre*. Seuil.

Roumain, Jacques. (1944) 2004. *Gouverneurs de La Rosée*. Mémoire d'Encrier.

Rowley, Michelle. 2002. "Reconceptualizing Voice: The Role of Matrifocality in Shaping Theories and Caribbean Voices." *Gendered Realities: Essays in Caribbean Feminist Thought*, edited by Patricia Mohammed, 22–43. Centre for Gender and Development Studies/University of the West Indes Press.

Sadai, Célia. 2009. "*D'eaux douces* de Fabienne Kanor: Triptyque cruel sur un corps insulaire." *La Plume Francophone*, April 2, 2009. http://la-plume-francophone.over-blog.com/article-29794601.html.

Salleh, Ariel. 1997. *Ecofeminism as Politics: Nature, Marx and the Postmodern*. Zed Books.

Schwarz-Bart, André. 1972. *La Mulâtresse Solitude*. Seuil.

Sharpe, Christina. 2016. *In the Wake: On Blackness and Being*. Duke University Press.

Sheller, Mimi. 2003. *Consuming the Caribbean from Arawaks to Zombies*. Routledge.

Siegal, Nina. 2015. "Rijksmuseum Removing Racially Charged Terms from Artworks' Titles and Descriptions." *New York Times*, December 10, 2015. https://archive.nytimes.com/artsbeat.blogs.nytimes.com/2015/12/10/rijksmuseum-removing-racially-charged-terms-from-artworks-titles-and-descriptions/.

Siqueira, Samanta Vitória, and Karine de Catilhos Lucena. 2020. "Aquela que diz não à sombra: Biografia e obra da escritora martinicana Françoise Ega." *Caligrama* 25 (3): 57–75. http://www.imigracaohistorica.info/uploads/1/3/0/0/130078887/aquela_que_diz_nao_a_sombra_siqueira_lucena.pdf.

Sol, Antoinette Marie. 2008. "Histoire(s) et traumatisme(s): L'infanticide dans le roman féminin antillais." *The French Review* 81 (5): 967–984. https://www.jstor.org/stable/25481325.

Snauwaert, Maïté, and Dominique Hétu. 2018. "Poétiques et imaginaires du *care*." *Temps Zéro* 12. http://tempszero.contemporain.info/document1650.

Spillers, Hortense J. 1987. "Mama's Baby, Papa's Maybe: An American Grammar Book." *Diacritics* 17 (2): 64–81. https://doi.org/10.2307/464747.

Thomas, Bonnie. 2017. "Gisèle Pineau: Writing as Therapy." *Connecting Histories: Francophone Caribbean Writers Interrogating Their Past*, 50–75. University Press of Mississippi.

———. 2021. "A Regarded Self: Caribbean Womanhood and the Ethics of Disorderly Being by Kaiama L. Glover." *L'Esprit Créateur* 61 (3): 146. https://doi.org/10.1353/esp.2021.0040.

Tronto, Joan C. 1993. *Moral Boundaries: A Political Argument for an Ethics of Care*. Routledge.

———. 2013. *Caring Democracy: Markets, Equality, and Justice*. New York University Press.

Tronto, Joan C., and Berenice Fisher. 1990. "Toward a Feminist Theory of Caring." *Circles of Care: Work and Identity in Women's Lives*, edited by Emily K. Abel and Margaret K. Nelson, 36–54. SUNY Press.

Trouillot, Evelyne. 2003. *Rosalie l'infâme*. Dapper.

Trouillot, Michel-Rolph. 1995. *Silencing the Past: Power and the Production of History*. Beacon Press.

Tsing, Anna. 2015. "Feral Biologies." Paper for Anthropological Visions of Sustainable Futures, University College London, Centre for the Anthropology of Sustainability (CAOS), University College London, February 13, 2015.

Tuck, Eve, and K. Wayne Yang. 2012. "Decolonization Is Not a Metaphor." *Decolonization: Indigeneity, Education and Society* 1 (1): 1–40. https://jps.library.utoronto.ca/index.php/des/article/view/18630.

Vergès, Françoise. 2011. *L'homme prédateur*. Albin Michel.

———. 2019a. "Capitalocene, Waste, Race, and Gender." *E-Flux*, no. 100. https://www.e-flux.com/journal/100/269165/capitalocene-waste-race-and-gender/.

———. 2019b. *Un féminisme décolonial*. La fabrique éditions.

Vété-Congolo, Hanétha. 2015. "Le couple nègre martiniquais, quel modèle: L'exemple de *D'eaux douces*." *Women in French Studies* 23 (1): 104–124. https://doi.org/10.1353/wfs.2015.0005.

Waller, Susan. (2006) 2017. *The Invention of the Model: Artists and Models in Paris, 1830–1870*. Routledge.

Weil, Simone. 1966. *Attente de Dieu*. Fayard.

Wimbush, Antonia. 2018. "Depicting French Caribbean Migration through Bande Dessinée." *International Journal of Francophone Studies* 21 (1): 9–29. https://doi.org/10.1386/ijfs.21.1-2.9_1.

———. 2022. "Madness, Isolation and the Female Condition in Gisèle Pineau's Writing." *Australian Journal of French Studies* 59 (2): 158–170. https://doi.org/10.3828/ajfs.2022.13.

Ziethen, Antje. 2012. "D'eutopie en dystopie: La poétique de l'espace antillais dans *Morne Câpresse* de Gisèle Pineau." *Nouvelles Études Francophones* 27 (2): 59–73. https://www.jstor.org/stable/24245214.

Zobel, Joseph. (1950) 2000. *La Rue Cases-Nègres*. Distribooks.

Notes on Cover Art

During a visit to the Freedom Monument Sculpture Park in Montgomery, Alabama, in March 2024, I encountered "The Caring Hand," a sculpture by Eva Oertli and Beat Huber. I remember pausing, deeply moved by how it evoked the interdependent relationship between individual and collective histories as well as living spaces, and the connection between human and nonhuman lives. The park, overlooking the Alabama River, houses historical artifacts of slavery and contemporary sculptures that collectively define an act of remembrance, honor the lives of enslaved and Indigenous people, and visually articulate the continuation of life. The hand, connecting to a tree grounded in the earth, symbolizes to me a gesture of retrieving humus from the soil, offering the possibility of restoration. There is also a sense of vulnerability in this bold gesture. Though scarred by the damage caused by the mortiferous systems of colonialism, enslavement, and the plantation, the rooted tree still continues to grow. The hand emerging from the earth and merging with the tree grasps not only the past buried deep within the ground but also willingly collects the seeds of change and reinvention. Through this hand, which connects to the tree—a metaphor for (re)growth—and to the earth, I see an invitation to engage in the act of healing our world, ourselves, others, and the lives long lost.

    I am grateful to Condé Nast, publisher of *The New Yorker*, for granting me permission to reproduce Kris Graves's photograph of

Eva Oertli and Beat Huber's sculpture. See Doreen St. Félix's article, "Bryan Stevenson Reclaims the Monument, in the Heart of the Deep South," published on March 25, 2024.

Index

Note: Page numbers in italics refer to illustrations.

Abenon, Lucien, and Jacques Cauna, *1789* (1989), 12
abolition, of slavery, 34, 41; of slave trade, 28
abuse, 8–9, 71, 76, 92–94, 96; emotional, 123; verbal, 154–155
accommodation, 71
Achard, Amédée, 38–39
Adrien (hospital patient), 153
adultery, 124–126, 142
Africa, 55; north, 39; South, 74; west, 27, 171n19
Africans, 27–44, 50, 55
Afro-Caribbean people, in Europe, 28–29, 36; in France, 31, 33–41, 57–88, 142. *See also* migration
Agnant, Marie-Célie, *Le livre d'Emma* (2002), 12
agriculture, 5, 22, 91, 94, 98, 104, 106, 113; ministry of, 114. *See also* gardening
Albert (uncle of Jessica Oublié), 78
Amaral, Claudia, 179n9
America: north, 27, 41, 104, 152; south, 5, 27, 41, 57, 125, 176n18
Amsterdam, Rijksmuseum, 35
Anacaona, Paula, and Claudia Amaral, *Solitude la flamboyante* (2020), 179n9
ancestry, 30, 92, 173. *See also* genealogy

André, Jacques, 132
Angélique (ancestor of Gisèle Pineau), 30
anonymity, 33, 36–38, 43, 46, 56, 76; deliberate, 68, 82. *See also* invisibility
Anselin, Alain, 58, 62–63
anthropologists, 34, 62–63, 105; Société d'Anthropologie de Paris, 39
Antillanité, 129
Antilles. *See* Caribbean
Arada people, 12
archives, 20, 43–46, 48, 53, 56, 80, 83, 86; Archives Départementales, Nantes, 44
aristocracy, 37, 49
art, visual, 28, 37–40; works of, 19, 29, 31, 33–34, 37–38. *See also* drawings
art: galleries, 35; schools, 36
artists, 36–37, 40. *See also individual artists*
asylums. *See* hospitals
attention, paying, 85–86, 88, 146, 151–152, 154–155, 158; hierarchy of, 21, 58, 65, 78
Avraam, Kathrine, 18, 22–23, 91, 104–117

Bachelard, Gaston, 74
Badagry (Nigeria), Door of No Return, 53
Baillif (Guadeloupe), 112
Bain turc ou maure (deux femmes) (Gérôme), 3
Baldwin, James, 1

bananas, 5, 22, 91, 104, 113, 180n11, 181n17, 183n22
bandes dessinées. *See* graphic narratives
Barbagallo, Camille, 61
Barthes, Roland, 15
Bazille, Frédéric, *La négresse aux pivoines*, now *Jeune femme aux pivoines* (1870), 35
beauty, 37, 40, 52
Bégué, Estelle, 38
Béké (white Creoles), 113, 182n22, 184n5
Benin, 171n19
Benjamin, Walter, *Arcades Project* (2003), 38
Benoît, Catherine, 105–106
Bernabé, Jean, 129
Bidou, Emmanuelle, and Fabienne Kanor, *Jambé dlo* (2008), 173n6
Bindman, David, *The Black Figure in the European Imaginary* (2017), 28, 40
biographies, 27, 32, 36; autobiographies, 145–159
bodies, materiality of, 46–49; racialized, 28, 93
Boni, Tanella, 112, 114, *115*
Bourdeau, Loïc, Natalie Edwards, and Steven Wilson, eds, "The Care (Re)turn in French and Francophone Studies" (2020), 13
Bourg, Dominique, 114, *115*
bourgeoisie, 37, 57–58, 66–70, 76
Boutrin, Louis, and Raphaël Confiant, *Chronique d'un empoisonnement annoncé* (2007), 5
Bratte, Emma (fictional character), 12
Brazil, 58
Britain, 28
Britton, Celia, 58
Brookes (slave ship), 28
Brugère, Fabienne, *Le sexe de la sollicitude* (2008), 139–140; *L'éthique du care* (2011), 2–3, 17
brutality, 159
Bureau pour le Développement des Migrations dans les Départements d'Outre-Mer (BUMIDOM), 20–21, 57–65, 68–70, 72, 75, 77–80, 82–83, 85, 88, 173n6
Bureau pour l'Installation des Personnes Immigrées en Guyane (Bipig), 176n18
Buste de nègre du Soudan (Cordier), 39

Calhoun, Doyle, 47–48
cancer, 106, *107*; International Agency for Research on Cancer, 5, 104
Câpresse (Cordier), 39
carcinogens, 5, 10, 22, 91, 104–108, 110–114, 180n11, 183n22
care, 1–2, 4, 6–11, 16–18, 25, 29, 42, 46, 54, 65–66, 80, 95, 103–104, 111, 122, 133, 146; ethic of, 7–8, 10, 16, 25–26, 100; negative, 8–9; rebellious, 23–24, 119–143; self-, 31, 128–130
caregivers, 43, 49–50, 58, 60, *64*, 65–66, 75–76, 88, 120, 145
caregiving, 13–16, 20–21, 23–26, 30–32, 36, 38–41, 45, 56, 61–62, 68–70, 74, 103, 121–122, 138–139, 143, 145, 147–155, 159
carelessness. *See* uncaring
care studies, 2, 13, 16, 18, 23, 25, 161
Caribbean, 1, 3, 5–6, 8–9, 11–13, 15, 17–18, 20–23, 25, 27, 40–41, 55, 57–59, 63, 65, 68, 70–72, 76, 78, 85–86, 89, 91, 94–96, 104–105, 145, 158–159
caring deficit, 7, 113
Carracci, Annibale, *Portrait of an African Woman Holding a Clock* (1583), 29
catastrophes, 103–104, 115
Cauna, Jacques, 12
caution, 124, 127
Célestine, Audrey, 58
Centre de Formation Professionnelle pour Adultes (or Centre d'Adaptation à la Vie Métropolitaine), 63
Césaire, Aimé, 5, 33, 166n5
Chabanne, Vivien, 35
Chamoiseau, Patrick, 129

204 Index

Chapon, Cécile, 89
Charon, Rita, "Narrative Medicine: A Model for Empathy, Reflection, Profession, and Trust" (2001), 152
chemicals, agricultural, 5, 10, 22, 91, 101, 104–108, 110–114, 180n11, 183n22
childcare, 38–40, 49–50, 68–70
children, 4, 6, 10–13, 28, 40, 74–76, 92, 96, 99, 102, 119, 123–124, 126, 158
Childs, Adrienne, 40
Chirac, Jacques, 34, 114
chlordecone, 5, 10, 22, 91, 101, 104–106, *107*, 108, 110–114, 180n11, 183n22
Christelle, Grande (fictional character), 136, 141–142
Christelle, Petite (fictional character), 136
Chute, Hillary, 78
citizenship, 3, 6, 86, *87*
Clarkson, Thomas, *History of the Rise, Progress, and Accomplishment of the Abolition of the African Slave Trade* (1808), 168n3
class, social, 2–3, 21, 37–38, 40–41, 60; struggle, 75, 137. *See also* aristocracy; bourgeoisie; working classes
Clérence, Faustina, 63
Cocteau, Jean, *La Belle et la Bête* (film, 1946), 174n9
coercion, psychological, 123
collectives: Care Collective, *The Care Manifesto* (2020), 7, 10; Kwazman Vwa, 111, 174n7, 182n19; Lyannaj kont' pwofitasyon, 6; Lyannaj pou dépolyé Matinik, 10, 112, 182n21
colonialism, 13, 17–23, 25, 29, 31, 34, 42–43, 61, 126, 145, 158
comic books. *See* graphic narratives
communities, female, 129–130; Congrégation des Filles de Cham (fictional community), 22, 91–104, 114, 116
compassion, 29, 155
Condé, Maryse, *La parole des femmes* (1979), 119

Condon, Stéphanie, 58
Confiant, Raphaël, 5, 129
confidence, 116–117, 136
consciousness, individual, 94
consignation, 45
consumers, 112
contamination. *See* pollution
cooking, 61, 76, 138
Cordier, Charles, *Buste de nègre du Soudan*, now *Homme du Soudan français* (1857), 39; *Câpresse* or *Négresse des colonies*, now *Femmes des colonies* (1861), 39; *Nègre du Soudan*, or *Nègre en costume algérien* (1856–1857), 40
couples. *See* lovers
courage, 23, 39, 126, 133. *See also* women: poto-mitan
COVID-19, 7
Créolité, 129
Cresson, Édith, 114
crimes, against humanity, 34. *See also* infanticide; murder
crops, 108. *See also* agriculture; bananas; gardening
Crouy-sur-Ourcq (Seine-et-Marne), 59, 62–63, *64*, 68
curation, 13, 15, 17–19, 29, 31–35, 42–43, 56
Curier, Charlise, *Mon aventure avec le BUMIDOM* (2019), 59–60, 62, 68
Curmer, Léon-Henri, ed., *Les français peints par eux-mêmes* (1840–1842), 38–39
Curtius, Anny Dominique, 58

Daisy (aunt of Gisèle Pineau), 30
daughters, 12, *69*, 123, 128, 131, 135, 138–143
deaths, 44, 48–49, 51–52, 121, 147, 149, 157
debauchery, 96
Débaury, Charles (fictional character), 92, 96
Debray, Cécile, 32–33
Debré, Michel, 57
decolonization, 1, 8–10, 14, 18

Degras, Priska, *L'obsession du nom dans le roman des Amériques* (2011), 41
dehumanization, 13, 28, 61, 74. *See also* individuality
DeLoughrey, Elizabeth, Renée Gosson, and George Handley, *Caribbean Literature and the Environment* (2005), 89–90
Démétrius, Madame (fictional character), 136, 142
Démétrius, Madeleine (fictional character), 24, 121, 132–135, 137, 141–142
Démétrius, Monsieur (fictional character), 142
democracy, 16, 100
depression, mental, 157. *See also* illness
Derrida, Jacques, 45
Deschênes, Marjorie, 14
desire, sexual, 135. *See also* lovers
Diallo, Rokhaya, and Grace Ly, "Kiffe ta race" (podcast, 2020), 113
diaries, 58–59, 60, 134
Diawara, Manthia, *Édouard Glissant: One World in Relation* (film, 2010), 105
disasters, 103. *See also* catastrophes
discretion, 71, 75, 132
disease, 55, 106, *107*
dispossession, 13, 27–29, 41, 52, 67, 93, 178
distress, 149
Divine (fictional character), 102
doctors. *See* medical personnel
documentaries, 59, 63, 105, 173n6
documents, historical, 42–46, 48, 53, 56, 79; personal, 29–30
domination, 41, 65, 74–76, 145; close, 67–68. *See also* oppression
Dorlin, Elsa, 8
drawings, 28, 111–113. *See also* art
Dufoix, Stéphane, 1

ecofeminism, 17, 94, 137, 178n6
École des Beaux-Arts (formerly the Académie des Beaux-Arts), Paris, 36, 37

Édouard (migrant), 80–82
education, secondary, 34; medical, 65
Edwards, Natalie, 13
Ega, Françoise, *Lettres à une Noire* (1978), 6, 18, 21, 57–58, 60–61, 66–67, 70–77, 79, 88; husband, 73
emotions, 147, 149–150, 155
empathy, 121, 133, 146, 152, 159
employers, 68–70. *See also* relationships
empowerment, 30, 74; disempowerment, 40, 94
Enfants aux Tuileries (Manet), 3
enslaved people, 28–29, 41–42, 44, 46–49, 52–56, 92, 105, 134, 136. *See also* slavery
environment, 21–22, 94–95, 103, 116; damage, 16–18, 21–22, 90–94, 98–99, 101, 104–105, 108, *109*, 110–112, 114, 116; restoration, 94; Environmental Protection Agency, U.S., 5
epidemiologists, 110
erasure, historical, 53. *See also* individuality
Eric (fictional character), 121–122, 124–126, 129
ethics, 35, 78, 91, 129; of care, 7–8, 10, 16, 25, 100
ethnography, 39–40
etymology, 45, 112, 156
Eunice (fictional character), 131, 137–139
exhibitions, 32; *L'Abîme* (Nantes, 2021–2022), 31; *Le modèle noir, de Géricault à Matisse* (Paris, 2019), 18–19, 29, 31, 33–34, 39, 42–43, 49, 56; *Le modèle noir, de Géricault à Picasso* (Guadeloupe, 2019), 19, 29, 33, 35, 38, 43, 56; *Marronnage* (Paris, 2022), 31
exit, from community, 97, 102
exoticism, 3, 90
exploitation, 6–8, 11–13, 18, 62, 72, 90, 92–93, 95, 98, 103, 178n6; of land, 21–22
exports, 113
expropriation, colonial, 95
extraction, 21, 90

fairy tales, 123–124
Falquet, Jules, 17
families, 73–78, 120, 122, 125–126, 138, 139–140, 154, 157–158; "antifamily," 125; nuclear, 123, 184n5
Fanon, Frantz, 93
farming. *See* agriculture; gardening
Federici, Silvia, 16, 61
feminism, 25. *See also* ecofeminism
Femmes des colonies (Cordier), 39
Ferdinand, Malcolm, 4, 114, *115*; *Une écologie décoloniale* (2019), 90, 97, 99
fertilizers, 98, 104
Feyen, Jacques-Eugène, *Le baiser enfantin* (1865), 40–41
fiction, 3–4, 6, 11–12, 15, 18–20, 23–24, 29–32, 41, 44–56, 90–104, 111, 120–124, 131–143
film, 59, 63, 174n9
fire, 103
Fisher, Berenice, 2, 9, 16, 130
Fleury, Cynthia, 114, *115*
Flore (fictional character), 12
Flore, Gilbert Jean Marie, 173n6
Flore, Ophélia Jean-Marie, 173n6
food, 76, 93, 105, 112, 138; organic, 102; supply, 22; vegan, 140
Fort-de-France (Martinique), 112–113, 172n4
Foucault, Michel, *History of Madness* (2013), 146
fragility, 13, 158–159
France, 3, 5–6, 8, 20, 24, 31, 34, 36–41, 57–63, 66–68, 71–72, 78, 80, 86, 92, 103, 121, 131–132, 135, 141–142, 145, 158, 181n18
Francis, Gladys M., *Odious Caribbean Women and the Palpable Aesthetics of Transgression* (2017), 46, 121, 124
Francky (nursing candidate), 157
Fred (gardener), 108, 110
freedom, of speech, 72; male, 125
French people, in Caribbean, 55
Frida (fictional character), 120–131, 143

friends, 24, 54, 78, 83, 121, 126, 132–133, 136, 141–142, 163
Fuentes, Marisa, 43, 52–53
fugitives, slave, 96–97. *See also* Maroons

gardening, 22, 66–67, 91, 95
Garden of Eden. *See* paradise
gardens, 156; *jardins créoles*, 91, 105–110; Jardins Familiaux (Jafa) program, 108. *See also* refuges
Gaspard (hospital patient), 153–154
Gefen, Alexandre, *Réparer le monde* (2018), 13–16, 42–43, 145, 151–152
gender, 2–4, 17, 21. *See also* men; women
genealogy, 30, 172–173n6
Géricault, Théodore, 36
Germain, Félix, 58
Gérôme, Jean-Léon, *Bain turc ou maure (deux femmes)* (1872), 3
Ghislaine (landowner), 108–110
Gilda (migrant), 83
Gilligan, Carol, *In a Different Voice* (1982), 2, 100
girls. *See* daughters
Gisèle (aunt of Gisèle Pineau), 30, 157
Glenn, Evelyn Nakano, 2, 10
Glissant, Édouard, 27, 96, 105–106, 111, 129, 136; *Le discours antillais* (1981), 89, 95, 125; *Le quatrième siècle* (1964), 41; *Poétique de la relation* (1990), 97. *See also* Diawara, Manthia
Glover, Kaiama, 128–130
Gobbi, Nicola, 18, 22–23, 91, 104–117
Gosier, Le (Guadeloupe), 63, 83
Gosson, Renée, 89–90
government, French, 20, 22, 59, 104
grandmothers, 122–123
graphic narratives, 1, 13, 15, 18, 21–22, 61, 68–70, 78–86, 91, 104–116
Guadeloupe, 1, 3–6, 10, 17, 20, 22, 24, 35, 57, 63, 77–78, 83, 89, 92, 102, 104, 112, 137, 145, 158–159, 165n5, 179n9, 180n13, 181n18
Guégan, Stéphane, 32–33

Index 207

Guérard, Henri, *Une Négresse, d'après Eva Gonzalès*, now *Jeune femme de profil (Laure?)*, *d'après Eva Gonzalès*, 33
Guiana, French, 5, 57, 125, 176n18
Gyssels, Kathleen, 125–126

habitat. *See* environment
Haiti, 3, 11–12, 36, 93
Handley, George, 89–90
Haraway, Donna, 4
Harpin, Tina, 95–96, 125
Hartman, Saidiya, "Venus in Two Acts" (2008), 30
healing, 55, 94; mental, 156; self-, 128, 130
health, 67, 71, 77, 91, 99, 106, *107*, 112, 114, 116, 136, 138, 141, 155–156; care, 24–25, 40; workers, 57. *See also* illness; nurses
Herbeck, Jason, 50
heritage, matrilineal, 122. *See also* genealogy
Hétu, Dominique, 154–155
hierarchy, institutional, 60, 68, 75, 98–100, 147–148, 150; racial, 28, 34, 44, 72; social, 37–38, 60, 72, 142. *See also* attention
Hirsch, Marianne, 78
Hirschman, Albert, *Exit, Voice, and Loyalty* (1970), 102
history, 19, 21, 43, 77–78, 89; colonial, 34–35, 50, 86, *87*; family, 30; oral, 79–86
Hochschild, Arlie, 16
home, sense of, 21, 72–76, 90, 100, 110, 112, 176n16
homemaking, 2, 73–75, 110
Homme du Soudan français (Cordier), 39
hooks, bell, "Homeplace: a site of resistance" (1990), 73–74
Hopewell (Virginia), 104
hospitals, 57, 71, 141; psychiatric, 145, 146–153, 155, 157–159
housekeepers, 71–73, 75, 142
husbands. *See* spouses

Ibos, Caroline, 61
illiteracy, 39
illness, 136, 138, 141; mental, 24, 146–147, 153, 155–157, 159
imports, 113
inattention. *See* uncaring
Indian Ocean, 5
individuality, erasure of, 13, 19–20, 29–30, 33–49, 54, 56; depersonalization, 62
infanticide, 11–12, 99, 124–126, 127, 130, 142
inhabitation, colonial, 21–22, 90, 92, 177n2
inheritance, 53–54
inhibitions, sexual, 132
insanity. *See* illness
insects. *See* weevils
interdependency, 67–68, 146
interiority, 151
interviews, 79–86
invisibility, 61–62, 75, 86, 100, 139, 146, 150, 153, 159
isolation, social, 67–68

Jackson, Laura, 146–147, 155
Jada (fictional character), 102
jardins créoles. *See* gardens
Jean-Charles, Régine Michelle, "Getting around the Poto-mitan" (2021), 135, 140; *Looking for Other Worlds: Black Feminism and Haitian Fiction* (2022), 25
Jessica (fictional character), 136
Jesus, Carolina Maria de, *Child of the Dark* (1960), 58, 72, 74–75, 77, 88
Jeune femme aux pivoines (Bazille), 35
Jeune femme de profil (Laure?), *d'après Eva Gonzalès* (Guérard), 33
José (landowner), 108–110
Joseph (artist's model), 36
Julia (grandmother of Gisèle Pineau), 30
justice. *See* social

Kanor, Fabienne, 173n6; *D'eaux douces* (2004), 18, 23–24, 120–132, 143; *Humus* (2006), 18–20, 29, 32, 44–56

Kepone. *See* chlordecone

killing, 11–12, 23, 52, 55, 99, 121, 124–130, 142, 147, 149, 157

Kincaid, Jamaica, 89

labor, 4, 6, 11, 16, 37, 44, 57, 59; domestic, 16–17, 40, 61, 63–65, 67–70, 72–76; migrant, 63, *64*; reproductive, 119; underpaid, 2, 40; unpaid, 2, 16; forced. *See* slavery

Lamour, Sabine, 133

landscape, 89, 116; damage, 21–22. *See also* environment

language, racist, 33–35; use of, 146, 154–157

Languedoc, 135, 141

Larose, Véronique, 122, 124

Larrier, Renée, 55

Laugier, Sandra, 2–3, 7–8, 11, 14, 17, 47, 52, 61, 65

Laure (servant), 33, 37

Lebrun, Vinciane, 18, 22–23, 91, 104–117

Lefaucheur, Nadine, "Situations monoparentales à la Martinique et idéal sacrificiel du potomitan" (2018), 120

legislation, 34; slave, 97; *Code Noir* (1685), 4, 27, 119

Léo (migrant), 83

Libby, Susan, 40

liberation, 11, 126–127, 129, 136; self-128–131, 143. *See also* Mouvement de Libération de la Négresse

Line (fictional character), 92–94, 97–103, 116–117

literature, 11, 13–16, 18, 22–25, 38–39, 46, 73, 90, 129, 146, 154–155

Loïc (fictional character), 133, 138

Loichot, Valérie, 156

Longin, Félix, *Voyage à la Guadeloupe* (1848), 180n13

Lorde, Audre, "The Transformation of Silence into Language and Action" (1984), 139

Louison, Monsieur (patient), 106

love, 51, 126; maternal, 11. *See also* romance

lovers, 23, 121, 124–129, 132, 135, 142, 158

Lucia, Soeur (fictional character), 99, 102

Lucienne, Saint, 134

Ly, Grace, 113

Macron, Emmanuel, 181n18

madness. *See* illness

Maestrati, Antoine-Léonard, *L'avenir est ailleurs* (film, 2007), 59, 63

maids, 76. *See also* servants

Manet, Édouard, *Enfants aux Tuileries* (c. 1861–1862), 3; *Olympia* (1863), 33, 37, 40–41

Mangangu, Bona, *Joseph Le Maure* (2016), 36

marginalization, 7, 14, 20, 40, 62, 70, 94, 100

Marine, Cellier, 89

Marlène (fictional character), 126

Maroons, 52, 91, 96–99, 179n9

marriage, 130. *See also* lovers

Marseille, 57–58, 62, 66–67, 72

Martial (migrant), 83

Martin, Laurent, 31–32

Martinique, 1, 3, 5–6, 10, 17, 20, 22, 24, 57, 66, 78, 80–82, 104, 121, 131–132, 141, 173n6, 181n18

masculinity, 126, 129; predatory, 124–126, 127; repressed, 184n7. *See also* men

matriarchy, 101, 183n3

Maximin, Daniel, *Les fruits du cyclone* (2006), 89

Mayotte, 5

McIlvanney, Siobhán, 146–147, 155

medical personnel, *64*, 65, 67, 71, 77, 152. *See also* midwives; nurses

medicine, 55. *See also* narrative

Mediterranean, 29

Memmi, Dominique, 67–68

Index 209

memoirs, 18, 30, 58–59
memory, 14, 20, 54–55, 171n19; suppression of, 60
men, 20, 23, 34, 36, 43–44, 51–52, 54–55, 57, 63–65, 73–74, 80–83, 92–93, 96, 119, 121, 123–127, 130–132, 135, 138, 142
messiahs, 99
Michel (farmer), 112
middle class. *See* bourgeoisie
Middle Passage, 27, 41, 89. *See also* slave trade
midwives, 12
Mignolo, Walter, and Catherine Walsh, *On Decoloniality* (2018), 9
migration, 6, 20, 40, 121; forced, 27–28; labor, 36, 57, 59–60, 63, *64*, 76, 80–86, 92
Milia-Marie-Luce, Monique, 85
Miller, Ann, 79–80
Milne, Lorna, 159
ministers, government, 114
minorities, 16, 31–32, 40, 79, 86, 88
Mitchell, Robin, *Vénus Noire* (2020), 36
models, artists', 33–34, 36–38, 40; Black, 19, 29, 32–35, 40, 43
Molinier, Pascale, Sandra Laugier, and Jules Falquet, *Genre et environnement* (2015), 17; with Sandra Laugier and Patricia Paperman, eds, *Qu'est-ce que le care?* (2009), 2–3, 7, 11, 61
Montpellier (Hérault), 35
morality, 2, 132
Morgan, Jennifer L., 29
Morne Câpresse (fictional location), 93, 96–100, 102, 116. *See also* Pineau, Gisèle
Mosnier, Louis, 44–45
motherhood, 11–13, 23, 58, 120; predatory, 123
mothers, 10–11, 122–124, 127, 130–131, 136–141, 158; "castrating", 123; overprotective, 124; "othermothers", 123
Mouvement de Libération de la Négresse (fictional organization), 128–129
Mulot, Stéphanie, 132, 137

Multigner, Luc, 110–111
murder, 12, 23, 99, 121, 124, 127–130, 143
Murdoch, H. Adlai, ed., *The Struggle of Non-Sovereign Caribbean Territories* (2021), 6, 58, 63
Murray, Cynthia Chantelle (fictional character), 132, 134–137, 139, 141
Murray-Román, Jeannine, 105–106, 108
Murrell, Denise, 32–33
museums, 35, 50; Musée Fabre, Montpellier, 35; Musée national d'Histoire naturelle, Paris, 40; Musée National de l'Histoire de l'Immigration, Paris, 88

Nallet, Henri, 114
names, abusive, 155; nicknames, 37, 41–43, 51, 73; personal, 32–33, 36–37, 41–43, 76; of works of art, 33, 35
nannies, 38–40, 49–50, 68–70
Nantes (Loire-Atlantique), 20
narrative: medicine, 152; voices, 70, 76–77, 79–80, 99, 126, 135
narratives, personal. *See* memoirs
National Assembly, French, 34
national identity, 86, *87*
nationalism, 137
natural resources, 16–17
Ndiaye, Pap, *La condition Noire* (2008), 58, 86, *87*
Neel (fictional character), 116–117
Nègre du Soudan (Cordier), 40
Nègre en costume algérien (Cordier), 40
Négresse, d'après Eva Gonzalès, Une (Guérard), 33
Négresse aux pivoines, La (Bazille), 35
Négresse des colonies (Cordier), 39
Nelson, Charmaine, *Representing the Black Female Subject in Western Art* (2010), 39–40
Nestor, Jacques, 165n5
Netherlands, 35
Ni Cheallaigh, Gillian, Laura Jackson, and Siobhán McIlvanney, eds, *Quand la folie parle* (2014), 146–147, 155

Nigeria, 53
Nina (fictional character), 131, 137–141
Noémie (nurse), 148–150
nonbeing, state of, 146
norms, social, 137, 142
novels, 3–4, 6, 11–13, 15, 18–20, 23–24, 29, 32, 41, 44–56, 90–104, 120–124, 131–143
nurses, 24, 40, *64*, 65, 146, 152–159; psychiatric, 145, 147–152; wet, 49–50. *See also* relationships
nurture, 29, 121

Oberhuber, Andrea, 14–16, 145, 150
Octavia, Gaël, *La bonne histoire de Madeleine Démétrius* (2020), 18, 24, 121, 131–143
officials, government, 113–114
Olympia (Manet), 33, 37, 40–41
oppression, 9, 11, 20, 41, 72, 74–75, 99, 101, 105, 122, 129–130, 133; patriarchal, 92–93
optimism, 116–117
Orlando, Natacha d', 89, 93, 95–96
Othering, 100, 113, 157–158; "Othercide," 177n2
Oublié, Jessica, 15; with Marie-Ange Rousseau, *Péyi an nou* (2017), 18, 21, 61–63, 68, 77–88; with Nicola Gobbi, Kathrine Avraam, and Vinciane Lebrun, *Tropiques toxiques* (2020), 18, 22–23, 91, 104–117
Ouidah (Benin), 171n19
Owens, Emily A., *Dispossessed Lives* (2016), 52

Pacôme, Sainte Mère (fictional character), 91–104, 116
painting, 3, 33. *See also* art; artists
Palermo, Lynn E., 54
pandemics, 7
papa-feuilles, 54–55
Paperman, Patricia, 2–3, 7, 11, 61
paradise, 90, 93–95
Paris, 34, 36–40, 71, 78, 80, 83, *84*, 86, 88, 131–132, 142

Paris Match (periodical), 58
pastimes, 149
patients. *See* relationships
Pattieu, Sylvain, 58
Pecresse, Valerie, 34
perception, 150–151
Persson, Ann-Sofie, 122
pesticides, 5, 10, 22, 91, 98, 101, 104–108, 110–114, 180n11, 181n17, 183n22
pests, insect, 5, 180n11
philosophers, 37, 38, 45, 47, 85
photography, 111–113
Pineau, Gisèle, 89; *L'exil selon Julia* (1996), 3–4; *Folie, aller simple* (2010), 24, 145–159; *Mes quatre femmes* (2007), 30–31; *Morne Câpresse* (2008), 18, 22–23, 90–104
Piovesan, Emmanuelle, 181n17
plantations, 4–5, 22, 93–94, 97–98, 104–105, 108, 125; "Plantationocene," 4
plants, medicinal, 55
Pludermacher, Isolde, 32–33, 38
Pointe-à-Pitre (Guadeloupe), 102
poisoning, 55
pollution, 10, 101, 104–106, 111; soil, 5, 105, 108–112; water, 5–6, 180n11
portraits, 37; *Portrait of an African Woman Holding a Clock* (Annibale Carracci), 29
poto-mitan. *See* women
poverty, 37, 58
power hierarchies, 18, 42, 68, 69
predators, sexual, 124–126
proletariat. *See* working classes
promiscuity, sexual, 124–126
property, humans as, 27–28, 44. *See also* slavery
protests, 165n5, 172n4, 181n18
proximity, 114, 150, 157–158

qualifications, 63–65

R., Sophie (hospital patient), 147–149
racism, 33–35, 39, 86, 154
Rancière, Jacques, 37

Index 211

rebellion. *See* resistance
recording devices, 79, 83–86
records, historical, 29–30, 37
recruitment, labor, 63–65, 68, 75–76
refuges, 150–151, 155–157
Régina, Soeur (fictional character), 101, 103
relations, social, 34, 72, 151–152
relationships, employer–worker, 68–72, 76–77; human–nonhuman, 16, 23, 89–91, 103, 110–112; patient–nurse, 147–153, 157; patient–physician, 152; sexual (*see* lovers)
religious belief, 141
Renaud, Leighan, 122–123
repression, 129, 136; matrilineal, 124; psychological, 123
reproduction, human, 4, 12, 178n6
Républicains, Les (political party), 34
resilience, 65, 119–120, 123, 133, 140
resistance, 12, 74, 76, 100, 126, 130, 165n5; slave, 20, 44, 46, 52, 91, 96–97, 99, 179n9
respectability, 132, 135, 137, 142
Returning, to Caribbean, 80, 92, 95
Réunion, 5, 20, 57, *84*
ritual, 96, 149–150
Rivière Salée (Martinique), 80–82
romance, 123–126. *See also* love
Rosalie (fictional character), 142
Roumain, Jacques, *Gouverneurs de la Rosée* (1944), 3
Rousseau, Marie-Ange, 18, 21, 61–63, 68, 77–78, *81*, 82, 85–86, *87*

Sadai, Célia, 122, 127
Saint-Claude (Guadeloupe), 158
Saint-Domingue. *See* Haiti
Saint-Maurice (Val-de-Marne), 145
São Paulo (Brazil), 58
schools, secondary, 34
sculpture, 39–40. *See also* art
secrecy, 59

self-: affirmation, 139; assertion, 72; awareness, 143, 146; censorship, 123; denial, 133; effacement, 122–123; expression, 52–53, 100, 129, 137, 141, 143; image, 132; presentation, 133; preservation, 51, 155; regard, 129; reliance, 93, 120; resignation, 120; sacrifice, 120; sufficiency, 106. *See also* care; healing; liberation
servants, 2–3, 6, 17, 28, 33, 37, 57–58, 60–70, 74–76, 122, 130, 142
shame, 59, 131, 136–137, 139, 142
Sharpe, Christina, *In the Wake* (2016), 25
ships, slave, 20, 27–28, 44, 52
sickness. *See* illness
silencing, 22, 28–32, 43–49, 53–54, 59–60, 95–96, 100, 122, 139, 150, 153. *See also* invisibility
Simandres (Rhône), 63, *64*
slaveholders, 42
slavery, 2–5, 9, 11–13, 18–21, 25, 27–31, 34, 42–43, 50–51, 53, 57, 61, 70, 89, 97, 119, 126, 143, 158, 179n9. *See also* enslaved people
slave trade, 12, 27, 53, 57, 171n19, 175n14
Snauwaert, Maïté, 154–155
social: hierarchy, 38, 40, 49, 72, 97–98; justice, 10, 14; media, 80, *81*, 111
sociology, 67, 120, 133, 137
soil, 81–82. *See also* pollution
Sol, Antoinette Marie, 11
soldiers, 132, 135
Le Soleil (slave ship), 44, 48, 52
Solitude, Mulâtresse, 137, 179n9
South Africa, 74
speaking, 47, 50; suppression of, 122. *See also* language
spouses, 138–139, 157–158; surveillance of, 127
stereotypes, gender, 65, 126–127, 133, 184n7; social, 39
storytelling, 79, 134

stress, mental, 150–151, 155–156
strikes, 165n5. *See also* protests
subalterns, 3, 16
subjugation, of women, 123. *See also* oppression
subsidies, agricultural, 112
suffering, 9, 12, 62, 94, 119, 123, 159
suicide, 44, 48–49, 52, 121, 128–129, 143, 147, 149, 157
Suzy (migrant), 83

teachers, 34–35, 63
Thomas, Bonnie, 156
Titi (migrant), *84*
titles. *See* names
Toly, Alex, 112
toxicity, 22, 113. *See also* carcinogens; chemicals
training, 62–63, 68
Trois-Rivières (Guadeloupe), 112
Tronto, Joan, *Moral Boundaries* (1993), 1–2, 9–10, 16, 113, 130
Trouillot, Evelyne, *Rosalie l'infâme* (2003), 11–12
Trouillot, Michel-Rolph, 34–35
trust, *69*, 121, 124, 127
Tsing, Anna, 4
Tuck, Eve, and K. Wayne Yang, "Decolonization Is Not a Metaphor" (2012), 9–10

uncaring, 5–8, 15, 17–18, 21, 25, 79, 88, 113–114, 158–159
unions, trades, 166n6
United States, 104, 152
universities, Sorbonne (Paris), 14
unrest, social, 59
utopianism, 95

vegetables, 108, *109*. *See also* food; gardening
verbality, 79–80. *See also* language
Vergès, Françoise, 4–5, 96–97
Vété-Congolo, Hanétha, 128

violence, 8, 12, 20, 22, 93, 98, 101, 103, 123, 129, 158; colonial, 48, 53, 56, 89, 94, 103; environmental, 23; maternal, 124; racial, 93
voice, individual, 51–52, 100, 102;
voicelessness, 47–48. *See also* self-: expression
vulnerability, 137–140, 146, 155, 158–159

Waller, Susan, *The Invention of the Model* (2006), 37
Walsh, Catherine, 9
watchfulness, 127
water supply, 22. *See also* pollution
weakness, 136, 138, 158
weevils, 5, 22, 91
Weil, Simone, 85
wellbeing, personal, 155
Wilson, Steven, 13
Wimbush, Antonia, 58, 158
wives. *See* spouses
womanhood, 123, 129, 131, 133, 135, 137, 142–143
women, 2–6, 10–12, 16–17, 20, 22, 28–30, 33, 37, 40, 43–76, 83, 91–103, 119–150, 179n9; *poto-mitan*, 23–24, 120–122, 129, 131–133, 136–137, 140–143
workers, health, 57; hospital, 147–148; indentured, 3; migrant, 38, 40, 62. *See also* labor
working classes, 36–37, 41
writers, 145–146, 149, 156–159; writer's block, 133–134
writing, 73, 75, 133–134, 136, 139–140, 150, 152–153, 155–156

X, Madame (hospital patient), 154

Yang, K. Wayne, 9–10
Yolande (maid), 66–67, 70–72

Ziethen, Antje, 95, 100
Zobel, Joseph, *La Rue Cases-Nègres* (1950), 3

Index 213

About the Author

JENNIFER BOUM MAKE is an assistant professor in the Department of French and Francophone Studies at Georgetown University. She is primarily a literary and visual studies scholar. Her research is focused on the French Caribbean, the legacy of colonialism and the French Atlantic slave trade, and care studies. Her scholarly work has been published in various venues, including *Nouvelles Études Francophones*, *Contemporary French and Francophone Studies*, and *Francosphères*, among others.

Available titles in the Critical Caribbean Studies series:

Giselle Anatol, *The Things That Fly in the Night: Female Vampires in Literature of the Circum-Caribbean and African Diaspora*

Alaí Reyes-Santos, *Our Caribbean Kin: Race and Nation in the Neoliberal Antilles*

Milagros Ricourt, *The Dominican Racial Imaginary: Surveying the Landscape of Race and Nation in Hispaniola*

Katherine A. Zien, *Sovereign Acts: Performing Race, Space, and Belonging in Panama and the Canal Zone*

Frances R. Botkin, *Thieving Three-Fingered Jack: Transatlantic Tales of a Jamaican Outlaw, 1780–2015*

Melissa A. Johnson, *Becoming Creole: Nature and Race in Belize*

Carlos Garrido Castellano, *Beyond Representation in Contemporary Caribbean Art: Space, Politics, and the Public Sphere*

Njelle W. Hamilton, *Phonographic Memories: Popular Music and the Contemporary Caribbean Novel*

Lia T. Bascomb, *In Plenty and in Time of Need: Popular Culture and the Remapping of Barbadian Identity*

Aliyah Khan, *Far from Mecca: Globalizing the Muslim Caribbean*

Rafael Ocasio, *Race and Nation in Puerto Rican Folklore: Franz Boas and John Alden Mason in Porto Rico*

Ana-Maurine Lara, *Streetwalking: LGBTQ Lives and Protest in the Dominican Republic*

Anke Birkenmaier, ed., *Caribbean Migrations: The Legacies of Colonialism*

Sherina Feliciano-Santos, *A Contested Caribbean Indigeneity: Language, Social Practice, and Identity within Puerto Rican Taíno Activism*

H. Adlai Murdoch, ed., *The Struggle of Non-Sovereign Caribbean Territories: Neoliberalism since the French Antillean Uprisings of 2009*

Robert Fatton Jr., *The Guise of Exceptionalism: Unmasking the National Narratives of Haiti and the United States*

Rafael Ocasio, *Folk Stories from the Hills of Puerto Rico/Cuentos folklóricos de las montañas de Puerto Rico*

Yveline Alexis, *Haiti Fights Back: The Life and Legacy of Charlemagne Péralte*

Katerina Gonzalez Seligmann, *Writing the Caribbean in Magazine Time*

Jocelyn Fenton Stitt, *Dreams of Archives Unfolded: Absence and Caribbean Life Writing*

Alison Donnell, *Creolized Sexualities: Undoing Heteronormativity in the Literary Imagination of the Anglo-Caribbean*

Vincent Joos, Urban Dwellings, *Haitian Citizenships: Housing, Memory, and Daily Life in Haiti*

Krystal Nandini Ghisyawan, *Erotic Cartographies: Decolonization and the Queer Caribbean Imagination*

Yvon van der Pijl and Francio Guadeloupe, eds., *Equaliberty in the Dutch Caribbean: Ways of Being Non/Sovereign*

Patricia Joan Saunders, *Buyers Beware: Insurgency and Consumption in Caribbean Popular Culture*

Atreyee Phukan, *Contradictory Indianness: Indenture, Creolization, and Literary Imaginary*

Nikoli A. Attai, *Defiant Bodies: Making Queer Community in the Anglophone Caribbean*

Samuel Ginsburg, *The Cyborg Caribbean: Techno-Dominance in Twenty-First-Century Cuban, Dominican, and Puerto Rican Science Fiction*

Linden F. Lewis, *Forbes Burnham: The Life and Times of the Comrade Leader*

Keja L. Valens, *Culinary Colonialism, Caribbean Cookbooks, and Recipes for National Independence*

Kim Williams-Pulfer, *Get Involved! Stories of Bahamian Civil Society*

Preity R. Kumar, *An Ordinary Landscape of Violence: Women Loving Women in Guyana*

Kezia Page, *Inside Tenement Time: Suss, Spirit, and Surveillance*

Natalie Lauren Belisle, *Caribbean Inhospitality: The Poetics of Strangers at Home*

Darlène Elizabeth Dubuisson, *Reclaiming Haiti's Futures: Returned Intellectuals, Placemaking, and Radical Imagination*

Elizabeth S. Manley, *Imagining the Tropics: Women, Romance, and the Making of Modern Tourism*

Jennifer Boum Make, *Decolonial Caregiving: Reimagining Caregiving in the French Caribbean*